Sleep

by Clete A. Kushida, MD, PhD

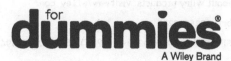

A Wiley Brand

Sleep For Dummies®

Published by: **John Wiley & Sons, Inc.**, 111 River Street, Hoboken, NJ 07030-5774, www.wiley.com

Copyright© 2025 by John Wiley & Sons, Inc. All rights reserved, including rights for text and data mining and training of artificial technologies or similar technologies.

Media and software compilation copyright © 2025 by John Wiley & Sons, Inc. All rights reserved, including rights for text and data mining and training of artificial technologies or similar technologies.

Published simultaneously in Canada

For general information on our other products and services, please contact our Customer Care Department within the U.S. at 877-762-2974, outside the U.S. at 317-572-3993, or fax 317-572-4002. For technical support, please visit https://hub.wiley.com/community/support/dummies.

Wiley publishes in a variety of print and electronic formats and by print-on-demand. Some material included with standard print versions of this book may not be included in e-books or in print-on-demand. If this book refers to media that is not included in the version you purchased, you may download this material at http://booksupport.wiley.com. For more information about Wiley products, visit www.wiley.com.

LLibrary of Congress Control Number: 2025933231

ISBN 978-1-394-26234-2 (pbk); ISBN 978-1-394-26236-6 (ePDF); ISBN 978-1-394-26235-9 (epub)

SKY10099230_030425

Contents at a Glance

Table of Contents

Introduction

Welcome to your handy reference guide to the fascinating and often misunderstood world of sleep! This book is your ticket to understanding everything from why people need sleep and how it works to the incredible technologies that can shape your night's sleep and the treatments that can transform lives for those who experience sleep issues.

Sleep impacts every aspect of your health, performance, and well-being — but it remains a mystery to many. By unlocking the secrets of sleep, you can gain the tools to achieve more restful nights, sharper days, and a deeper appreciation for this essential part of life.

I wrote this book with the curious beginner in mind, packing it with expert insights, practical advice, and real-life examples to keep the content relevant and engaging. So grab your favorite blanket, settle in, and get ready to embark on a journey to better sleep and better health!

About This Book

Although no shortage of advice on sleep exists, this book stands apart as a thorough introduction to understanding, improving, and appreciating sleep as a vital part of life. It's your go-to resource for exploring the science of sleep, tackling common or rare sleep disorders, and making changes to achieve your best rest yet. With fascinating insights into how sleep works, actionable advice for healthier habits, and the latest technologies in sleep science, this book can help you turn good intentions into truly restorative nights.

Like all For Dummies books, this one is organized to make finding the information you need simple and quick. I've divided it into five parts:

>> **Part 1 dives into the foundations of sleep** and covers its stages, how it changes with age, why it's essential, and the science behind it.

>> **Part 2 takes a deeper look at how sleep interacts with the body's systems,** from the nervous system to circadian rhythms, and even explores the mystery of dreams.

>> **Part 3 is packed with practical advice** for overcoming sleep deprivation, seeking expert help, managing disorders, and building healthy sleep-related habits.

>> **Part 4 focuses on the tools and technologies** that reshape sleep health, from sleep lab diagnostics to wearable devices and cutting-edge treatments.

>> **Part 5 distills key insights into quick, easy-to-reference lists.** Whether your goal is to explore, troubleshoot, or transform your sleep, this book is your trusted companion.

Foolish Assumptions

Whether you're struggling with sleepless nights, curious about the science of sleep, or looking for practical tips to improve your shut-eye, this book is here to guide you. It's designed to help everyone — from the occasional napper to the chronically sleep-deprived — find solutions that work for their unique situation.

And I do make a few assumptions about you and your situation:

>> **You may be picking up this book because you want to sleep better,** improve your alertness during the day, or optimize your overall health.

>> **You may be reading this book for someone else's benefit.** Maybe your child has trouble sleeping through the night, your partner's snoring is keeping you up, or you're trying to support a loved one with a challenging sleep disorder.

   If that sounds like you, this book has plenty of advice to help you understand what they're going through and what steps you can take to help both of you get the rest you deserve.

>> **You aren't medical professionals** (most of you, that is), and that's okay. This book breaks down sleep science in a way that's easy to understand, even if you don't have a background in health or medicine.

   That said, for those of you who are especially curious or happen to know a bit more about the subject, I've included some technical deep dives.

>> **You agree that sleep is essential to living your best life.** It's not just about avoiding exhaustion — it's about waking up energized, thinking clearly, and thriving during the day.

My goal is to make this book an inclusive and supportive resource, offering you practical advice, expert insights, and encouragement as you work toward better nights and brighter mornings.

Icons Used in This Book

Throughout this book, you may notice icons in the margins that highlight key points or essential advice. These icons are here to make finding the most valuable nuggets of information easy to do while you read. Here's what each icon means.

The *Tip* icon points out helpful hints and insider advice that can make improving your sleep even easier. Think of it as your friendly sleep coach offering quick, actionable ideas to make your nights (and days) better.

The *Remember* icon highlights information that's especially important to keep in mind. If you're short on time, these icons help you zero in on the most critical must-know details about sleep and how it affects you.

Occasionally, as I mention in the preceding section, I use the *Technical Stuff* icon to highlight a bit of deeper knowledge regarding the science of sleep or its treatment. If that's not your gig, feel free to avoid the material marked by these icons.

The *Warning* icon is there to help you avoid potential pitfalls or hazards. Always take note of these! Whether it's about avoiding a bad habit that harms your sleep or being cautious with certain treatments, this icon keeps you and your sleep on the right track.

Beyond the Book

In addition to the wealth of sleep information and guidance in this book, you have access to even more resources online at Dummies.com. Be sure to check out this book's online Cheat Sheet for quick, handy insights into the basics of sleep. You can find high-level summaries of sleep architecture (states and stages), snapshots of six major sleep disorders (such as insomnia and sleep apnea), and a list of healthy sleep tips to help you improve your nightly routine.

To access the Cheat Sheet, simply visit www.dummies.com, type *sleep for dummies cheat sheet* in the search box, and click the search icon. It's a great way to keep essential sleep knowledge at your fingertips!

Where to Go from Here

This book is here to meet you exactly where you are — whether you're exhausted, frustrated, or simply curious about sleep. The best part? You don't have to read it from cover to cover to find what you need. Each chapter stands on its own, so you can jump right to the information that speaks to your situation.

REMEMBER

Of course, you can always review the Table of Contents to find chapters or sections of particular interest. And the Index gives you another excellent way to locate topics that you need to know about.

If you're worried about a sleep disorder — whether it's insomnia, sleep apnea, or something more unusual — flip to Chapters 7 and 8 for expert guidance on recognizing symptoms and understanding treatments. Struggling to get your child, partner, or even yourself to sleep soundly? Chapter 6 is full of practical tips for improving sleep routines at any age. If you're wondering how technology might help (or hurt) your sleep, Chapter 11 gives you the lowdown on the latest gadgets and how to use them wisely. And if you just want quick ways to improve your sleep, Chapter 15 provides easy-to-follow tips that can make a big difference fast.

No matter what caused you to seek sleep information and help, this book has you covered. Take a deep breath — you're in the right place, and you're not alone.

1

Getting Started with Sleep Basics

Chapter 1

Exploring Sleep's Fundamental Nature

Every night, billions of people close their eyes, surrendering to a state that has puzzled and fascinated scientists, philosophers, and poets alike for centuries: sleep. For something so universal, sleep remains one of the most complex and poorly understood processes of the human body. Sleep is not just a nightly shutdown; it involves a complex dance of chemical messengers from the brain that interact with biological rhythms. Sleep is a vital activity that underpins all bodily processes — from memory to immunity.

This book unravels the questions of sleep by diving into its science, challenges, and solutions. As someone who has dedicated decades to studying this field, I've witnessed firsthand the profound impacts of both healthy and disordered sleep. Whether you examine the devastating consequences of chronic sleep deprivation or the life-changing effects of a good night's rest, one aspect is clear: Sleep matters. It matters for your health, your productivity, and your happiness.

Sleep's role in people's lives is more crucial now than ever. Modern life — with its constant barrage of screens, deadlines, and stress — has turned sleep into an elusive commodity. For many people, getting the recommended seven to nine hours of sleep feels like a distant dream that's been replaced by exhaustion and caffeine-fueled mornings.

In this chapter, I walk you through the fundamentals of sleep — what it is, why it's essential, and how it changes throughout our lives. I also touch on the fascinating world of sleep science, disorders, and optimization. This chapter helps you see sleep not as a passive downtime, but as a powerful tool for transformation.

Understanding the Composition of Sleep

Sleep may feel like a single continuous experience, but beneath the surface, sleep harbors an intricate symphony of biological activity. From the gentle transitions of light sleep to the vivid dreams of REM sleep, every stage plays a unique role in restoring your body and mind.

Stages and states of sleep

When you fall asleep, your brain doesn't simply turn off. Instead, it moves through two distinct states: Non-Rapid Eye Movement (NREM) sleep and Rapid Eye Movement (REM) sleep.

NREM sleep forms the foundation of restorative sleep and dominates most of the sleep cycle. It consists of three stages that serve unique purposes and repeat in cycles throughout the night:

>> **Stage N1:** This is the gateway to sleep — a light, transitional stage marked by slower brain waves (like theta waves at 5–7 Hz versus alpha waves at 8–12 Hz, which dominate the wake state). Your muscles relax and eye movements slow down. People often don't realize they're asleep during this stage.

>> **Stage N2:** Often called *intermediate sleep*, this stage makes up 40 to 55 percent of your nightly rest. It features hallmark brain wave patterns — including sleep spindles and K-complexes — which help consolidate memories and suppress external stimuli.

>> **Stage N3:** Also known as *slow-wave sleep* or *deep sleep*, this stage is essential for physical recovery. During the N3 stage, your body repairs tissues, clears brain toxins, and strengthens the immune system.

Turn to Chapter 2 for more information about each stage of NREM sleep.

After NREM, you enter the state of REM sleep, which occurs about 90 minutes after you fall asleep and recurs multiple times throughout the night. Each period of REM sleep grows longer. During REM, your brain activity mimics wakefulness, but your body remains in a state of temporary paralysis. During this sleep stage, the majority of your dreams occur, and experiencing it is critical for emotional regulation and memory consolidation.

REMEMBER

Sleep specialists often refer to REM sleep as a *state* rather than a *stage* of sleep because it is so different from NREM stages of sleep.

Altogether, the states and stages of sleep form a roughly 90-minute cycle that repeats four to six times during an average night. Each cycle shifts in composition as the night progresses, with deep sleep (N3) dominating earlier cycles and REM sleep taking over later on. Visit Chapter 2 to read more about sleep stages and states.

While sleep stages are universal, the way people cycle through them can vary. For example,

>> **Genetics** may play a role in determining your natural sleep tendencies, including whether you're a morning lark or a night owl. See Chapters 7 and 8 for additional information on the role of genetics in sleep disorders.

>> **Lifestyle factors,** such as exercise, diet, and stress levels, also influence how easily your body transitions through sleep stages. A sedentary lifestyle may contribute to lighter, more fragmented sleep, and consistent physical activity promotes deeper slow-wave sleep. See Chapter 6 for information about how your lifestyle and habits affect your sleep.

>> **Aging** causes the way your body navigates through sleep stages to change naturally. Newborns need more sleep (of varying stages) than do older humans, who spend less time in deep sleep and more time in the lighter stages.

>> **External factors,** such as medications, stress situations, sleep disorders, or the makeup of your sleep environment all have an effect on the quality and quantity of your sleep.

REMEMBER

Sleep specialists and researchers don't really know which sleep states and stages are most critical to overall health. But from certain studies on animals and humans, they know that deeper stages of sleep and REM sleep are particularly important, and that sleep deprivation for lighter stages of sleep does not have as substantial an effect.

And although sleep specialists can identify the stages and states of sleep, they don't know why people sleep. But I do cover a few prevailing theories about the reason for sleep in Chapter 2.

Sleep components and characteristics

During sleep, your conscious mind takes a break, but your body and brain perform critical maintenance that supports your health and well-being. Sleep is marked by distinct neurophysiological and physical changes, all of which help restore your energy and optimize your body's functions. I cover these aspects of sleep in detail in Chapter 4, but here's a quick glance at them:

>> **Circadian system:** Your sleep-wake cycle is largely controlled by your sleep drive and by your circadian sleep-wake rhythm, which follows a roughly 24-your cycle. One of the strongest influences on this rhythm is light. Exposure to light in the morning can allow you to wake up earlier, and evening light can delay the onset of sleep.

>> **Dreams:** Most dreaming occurs during REM sleep, when the brain is highly active, particularly in the limbic system, which governs emotions. Dreams play a role in emotional processing, learning, and even simulating waking-life scenarios. Dreams also reflect the activity in regions of the brain associated with vision and emotion, which can make dreams richly sensory and often emotionally intense. Interestingly, dream recall happens primarily when you briefly wake during or after REM sleep, which is a natural part of nightly cycles. Flip to Chapter 5 for a breakdown of theories on dreaming.

>> **Effects on body systems:** During the transition from wakefulness to light sleep, your breathing changes as it switches from conscious control to an autonomic mechanism, and during REM sleep, your breathing becomes shallower and irregular. Similarly, other body systems react, including

   - *Your heart rate and blood pressure* can fluctuate during REM sleep.

   - *Your digestive system* undergoes a change, with gastric acid secretion peaking in the early morning hours, and during REM sleep, your digestion is generally more active.

   - *Growth hormone secretion* surges during deep NREM sleep, promoting repair and growth of tissues.

   - *Body temperature* varies during sleep, and during REM sleep, your body can't regulate temperature as efficiently, leading to unpredictable swings in temperature.

   Head to Chapter 3 for all of the ways sleep impacts your body.

>> **Differences due to sex:** Women tend to sleep longer than men, and differences in EEG activity between women and men occur during the sleep stages. Additionally, sleep disturbances are common during pregnancy, postpartum, and menopause. Turn to Chapter 6 to discover more differences in sleep between men and women.

>> **Neurotransmitters:** These chemical messengers play a role in regulating NREM and REM sleep. For example, GABA (gamma-aminobutyric acid) is an inhibitory neurotransmitter that slows down brain activity and helps induce sleep, and orexin (hypocretin) stabilizes wakefulness and prevents transitions to sleep.

>> **Racial and ethnic differences:** Racial minorities are more likely to experience sleep disruptions and shorter sleep durations, and cultural practices vary among ethnic groups with respect to co-sleeping and napping. Turn to Chapter 6 for more details on how sleep differs across race and ethnicity.

>> **Wake-sleep and sleep-stage regulation:** A group of nuclei in the brainstem plays a major role in the promotion of sleep and wakefulness, and also in alternating NREM and REM sleep. If the balance of the neurotransmitters in the brainstem is off, you can experience disorders of excessive sleep (such as narcolepsy) or too little sleep (such as insomnia).

Changes in sleep, movement, and behavior during the night

Your body undergoes a dynamic array of changes as it transitions between sleep stages and cycles. These changes in heart rate, brain activity, and even physical movements are critical to your body's restorative processes:

>> **Body movements:** While you may shift positions or adjust your blanket during lighter stages of sleep (like N1 and N2), your body becomes more relaxed as you transition into deeper stages. This relaxation conserves energy and promotes recovery. On the other hand, disorders such as restless legs syndrome (RLS) or REM sleep behavior disorder (RBD) disrupt this stillness and can lead to excessive or even dangerous movements during the night. To learn more about these conditions, explore the detailed discussion in Chapter 8.

>> **Brain activity and dreaming:** Your brain stays busy while you sleep. Deep sleep (N3) is a time for synchronized delta waves, which help your brain strengthen memories and recover from the day's demands. As the night progresses and REM sleep takes over, dreaming is more likely to occur, and activity ramps up in brain areas tied to emotions and creativity. If you're curious about the fascinating science behind dreams, check out Chapter 5.

>> **Heart rate and breathing:** Your cardiovascular and respiratory systems respond to the demands of each sleep stage. In deep sleep (N3), your heart rate and breathing slow and become regular (when compared to the wake state), creating the perfect conditions for physical repair. Chapter 4 sheds light on how these systems function together and how sleep disruptions can impact your health.

>> **Hormonal shifts:** Hormones work behind the scenes to keep your body in balance while you sleep. Growth hormone peaks during deep sleep, repairing tissues and supporting muscle recovery, while cortisol — your primary stress hormone — dips to its lowest levels early in the night. This delicate hormonal choreography prepares you for both physical restoration and the challenges of the next day. Flip to Chapter 4 for an in-depth look at how sleep influences your hormonal health.

>> **Temperature regulation:** Sleep also impacts how your body handles its internal temperature. During NREM sleep, your core temperature naturally drops, which helps you stay comfortable and enter deeper stages of rest. During REM sleep, however, your body's temperature regulation turns off, leaving you more vulnerable to external factors like a hot or chilly room. A bedroom set to a cool 60–67 degrees F can help you maintain comfort throughout the night. For additional tips on creating the ultimate sleep sanctuary, turn to Chapter 3.

TIP

If you wake up frequently feeling overheated, try adjusting your room's temperature or swapping out heavy blankets for breathable, lightweight options. Small changes to your environment can make a big difference.

These nightly changes are part of the body's intricate design to promote health and restoration, but disruptions may throw these processes off balance, leaving you feeling groggy and unfocused the next day. Chapter 3 offers tips for managing environmental factors to create an optimal sleep setting. Also, Chapter 6 gives you the scoop on how lifestyle choices such as diet, stress management, and alcohol use affect your sleep quality.

REMEMBER

If you experience repeated disruptions to sleep cycles — whether because of lifestyle factors or medical conditions — you may see long-term impacts on your physical and mental health. If you experience persistent sleep difficulties, consult a healthcare professional for personalized advice and solutions. In Chapter 9, you can find out about seeking help for sleep issues, and Chapters 10 and 11 give you a look at how technology — in a sleep clinic or at home — can help with diagnosis and treatment of sleep problems.

Discovering Sleep as a Lifelong Activity

How people sleep — and how much sleep they need — changes dramatically as they grow and age. These shifts are not random; they reflect the evolving demands of our bodies and brains during different life stages. Understanding these changes can help you adjust your routines and expectations, ensuring that you get the best possible sleep at every age.

Sleep begins to shape human lives from the moment of birth, playing a vital role in growth, development, and overall well-being. In this section, you get a glimpse of how sleep evolves across the human lifespan, and what you can do to nurture sleep for yourself and other family members. For more information about sleep at various life stages, check out Chapter 6.

For babies and children

Few things are more associated with early life than the image of a peacefully sleeping baby. Sleep during infancy is critical for brain development because, while babies sleep, their brains form millions of new neural connections and begin to consolidate early experiences. Newborns need between 16 and 18 hours of sleep per day, but their sleep occurs in short bursts of two to four hours throughout the day and night due to their immature circadian rhythms.

By six months of age, most babies can sleep for longer stretches at night, with naps during the day becoming more structured. Preschoolers and school-aged children need around 9–12 hours of sleep nightly to support growth, memory, and emotional regulation. However, external factors like busy schedules, screen time, and environmental distractions often interfere. To foster healthy sleep habits:

>> **Create comfort.** Ensure your child's bedroom has a cozy, quiet environment with the right temperature and supportive bedding.

>> **Encourage consistency.** Set a regular bedtime and wake-up time to establish a routine.

>> **Limit screen time.** Avoid electronic devices at least an hour before bed, because mental activity is not conducive to sleep, and the blue light can interfere with melatonin production.

>> **Set a bedtime routine.** Calming activities like reading, bathing, or listening to soft music help signal that it's time for sleep.

WARNING

Children who don't get enough sleep often show symptoms like irritability, hyper-activity, or trouble concentrating. These behaviors can mimic ADHD, so it's crucial to rule out sleep deprivation as a contributing factor.

For adolescents

Teenagers face unique challenges related to sleeping. Biological changes during puberty delay the release of melatonin, the hormone that promotes sleep, which makes falling asleep early at night harder for teens to do. Although they still need eight to ten hours of sleep nightly, situations such as late-night screen use, social pressures, and early school start times often leave teenagers sleep-deprived.

The effects of sleep deprivation in teens are far-reaching and include difficulty focusing, mood swings, and even increased risk-taking behaviors. To help teens get better sleep, you can

>> **Advocate for a consistent schedule.** Encourage teens to maintain a regular bedtime and wake-up time, even on weekends.

>> **Encourage sleep-friendly environments.** Ensure their bedroom is cool, dark, and quiet.

>> **Establish screen boundaries.** Limit digital-device use at least an hour before bed.

>> **Promote a wind-down routine.** Help teens relax with calming activities like reading or journaling.

WARNING

Chronic sleep deprivation during adolescence can increase the risk of anxiety, depression, and even car accidents due to drowsy driving.

For adults

Life as an adult often feels like a juggling act. Between work, family, and personal responsibilities, sleep is often one of the first sacrifices. But adults need seven to nine hours of sleep per night to function optimally. Chronic sleep deprivation is linked to a host of health problems, including impaired memory, weight gain, and increased risk of heart disease. To claim better sleep, you can

>> **Establish boundaries with technology.** Avoid checking emails or scrolling social media close to bedtime.

>> **Invest in sleep-friendly spaces.** Optimize your bedroom with supportive bedding, blackout curtains, and a comfortable mattress.

>> **Make sleep a priority.** Treat rest as a nonnegotiable part of your health routine.

>> **Practice a bedtime routine.** Include activities like light stretching, meditation, or listening to calming music.

TIP

If you frequently wake up tired despite spending enough time in bed, you may need to adjust your sleep environment. See Chapter 15 for practical tips on optimizing your sleep space.

For older adults

As people age, sleep often becomes lighter and more fragmented. Seniors may find themselves waking more frequently during the night or needing naps during the day. These changes are partly due to shifts in circadian rhythms, as well as health conditions or medications that can interfere with rest. Despite these challenges, older adults still need seven to eight hours of sleep per night to maintain good health. To get better sleep in later life, try

>> **Addressing your health concerns.** Speak with a healthcare provider about conditions such as chronic pain or medications that may affect your sleep. Your provider can also help to identify serious sleep problems that might need a referral to a sleep specialist.

>> **Establishing a calming bedtime routine.** Gentle stretching, warm baths, or listening to soothing music can help signal your body to wind down.

>> **Staying active during the day.** Regular physical activity promotes deeper sleep at night.

WARNING

Many older adults believe poor sleep is just part of aging, but recognizing when an underlying issue might be at play is important. If left unaddressed, sleep problems can lead to an increased risk of falls, memory difficulties, and significant mood changes.

Focusing on Your Need for Sleep

Busy people in the modern world often dismiss sleep as a luxury in today's fast pace. But the need for sleep is as fundamental as the need for food or water. When you neglect healthy sleep, the effects ripple through every part of your life — your health, productivity, and even your safety. Understanding why sleep matters starts with recognizing its role in restoring your body and mind and distinguishing between related issues like sleepiness and fatigue.

Sleepiness versus fatigue

At first glance, sleepiness and fatigue might seem like the same thing, but they're distinct experiences with different causes. Sleepiness is your body's way of signaling that it needs rest, and it's often caused by insufficient sleep or disruptions in your sleep cycle. Sleepiness is the drowsy feeling you get when your eyelids feel heavy and your ability to focus diminishes.

Individuals with sleepiness can't stay awake, especially in situations such as participating in a meeting or while reading. Fatigue, on the other hand, goes beyond the desire to sleep. It's a deeper, lingering exhaustion that can persist even after a full night's rest. Fatigue often stems from underlying medical conditions — chronic fatigue syndrome, for example — or lifestyle factors such as stress and poor nutrition. Addressing fatigue may require more than just improving your sleep; it often involves a holistic approach to health and well-being.

Distinguishing between sleepiness and fatigue is particularly important for managing your condition successfully, so always do your best to convey your symptoms accurately to your healthcare provider.

If you regularly feel tired despite sleeping enough, consider keeping a sleep log or sleep diary. (See Chapter 9 for details on keeping a sleep diary.) When you do, you can track your sleep patterns, energy levels, and lifestyle habits to identify potential triggers. Share anything that seems concerning with your doctor to see whether you may need a sleep study.

Sleepiness as an epidemic

Sleepiness has become a societal epidemic, fueled by modern habits and a culture that glorifies busyness. The rise of technology, with its endless stream of notifications and bright screens, has led to widespread sleep deprivation, according to several research studies, especially in young adults. Work schedules, commuting, and 24/7 connectivity have created a world in which many people simply don't get enough rest. The result? A population that is perpetually running on empty.

Chronic sleepiness affects more than just individuals — it has a societal cost. Various research findings link sleep deprivation to increased rates of accidents, errors at work, and chronic illnesses such as heart disease and diabetes. In fact, drowsy driving contributes to thousands of traffic accidents each year — for example, approximately 91,000 annually according to in-depth crash investigations conducted for the National Highway Traffic Safety Administration (reported in the 2024 research brief "Drowsy Driving in Fatal Crashes, United States, 2017–2021") by the American Automobile Association (AAA) Foundation for Traffic Safety at https://aaafoundation.org.

The National Transportation Safety Board (NTSB) has also reported an increase in traffic accidents associated with the shift in schedules for daylight savings time — both in the spring and fall — due to disturbed sleep patterns that lead to increased driver sleepiness.

Recognizing sleepiness as a public health issue is the first step toward addressing it. Employers, schools, and policymakers can play a role by promoting healthier work-life balance, encouraging flexible schedules, providing time and space for napping (especially for those diagnosed with narcolepsy), and educating the public about the importance of rest. (See Chapter 3 for more on how sleep impacts workplace performance and safety.)

Sleepiness in diverse occupations and environments

The consequences of sleepiness vary depending on your environment and work responsibilities, but certain professions are especially vulnerable. Healthcare workers, for example, often work long, irregular shifts, which makes them prone to burnout and errors. Professional drivers and transportation and safety workers face high stakes because even a momentary lapse in attention can result in tragedy. Creative professionals, meanwhile, may underestimate how critical rest is for sustaining innovative thinking and problem-solving skills.

REMEMBER

Regardless of your profession or setting, keep yourself and others safe by

>> **Optimizing your environment.** Ensure your workspace has good lighting, comfortable seating, and minimal distractions to support alertness.

>> **Prioritizing rest.** Build breaks and recovery periods into your schedule, especially during demanding work cycles.

>> **Recognizing limits.** Know when it's time to step away from tasks that require high concentration if you're feeling drowsy.

For those in high-risk professions such as healthcare or transportation and safety, advocate for institutional changes — such as reduced shift lengths or mandatory rest periods. These measures help create safer environments for everyone.

Knowing the Characteristics of Healthy Sleep

Healthy sleep isn't just about how long you sleep (the quantity), but it's also about the quality. Sleep that restores your body and mind has specific characteristics, and understanding these can help you assess whether you're truly getting both the quantity and the quality of sleep you need. While everyone's sleep needs vary slightly, some universal markers of healthy sleep apply across all ages. Healthy sleep has three main components that together create the foundation for feeling refreshed and alert during the day:

>> **Continuity:** Having enough sleep is important, but so is having uninterrupted sleep. Healthy sleep should occur in one consolidated block, without frequent awakenings. Fragmented sleep — even if the total hours add up to a sufficient amount — reduces your time in restorative stages such as deep sleep and REM. (For more on sleep stages, you can refer to the section "Understanding the Composition of Sleep" earlier in the chapter and also to Chapter 2.)

>> **Depth:** The intensity of sleep, particularly during deep sleep (slow-wave sleep), is critical for physical recovery and memory consolidation. While you may not be able to measure sleep depth directly at home, you can assess it by how refreshed you feel upon waking. People who regularly experience shallow or disrupted sleep often wake up groggy, with lingering fatigue.

>> **Duration:** The National Sleep Foundation (at www.thensf.org) recommends seven to nine hours of sleep per night for adults, with slight variations depending on individual needs. Children and teens require more because their developing bodies and brains rely heavily on restorative rest. Sleeping consistently within your recommended range is one of the most important steps toward maintaining overall health.

The role of circadian rhythms

Healthy sleep is deeply tied to your *circadian rhythms* — the internal biologic clock that regulates your sleep-wake cycle. These rhythms are influenced by natural light and darkness, which signal your body to release sleep-promoting hormones like melatonin. Aligning your schedule with these rhythms can improve the quality of your life.

>> **Evening habits:** Dim the lights in your home as bedtime approaches, and avoid blue light from screens. These behaviors may impact melatonin signals to your body that it's time to wind down.

>> **Morning routines:** Expose yourself to natural light within the first hour of waking. This practice helps regulate your circadian rhythms and promotes alertness during the day.

For those who struggle with circadian misalignment — such as shift workers or frequent travelers (who cross time zones) — establishing consistent sleep routines and using tools such as light therapy devices can help reset your internal clock. Flip to Chapter 8 for strategies tailored to circadian rhythm challenges.

TIP

Struggling to make changes? Start small. Focus on one aspect of your sleep, such as your bedtime routine, and gradually build from there. Consistency is more important than perfection.

Nutrition, exercise, and sleep

Getting good nutrition and regular exercise are essential for maintaining healthy sleep. Here are some general guidelines regarding eating and drinking:

>> **Eat foods rich in unsaturated fats and high in fiber** to help promote deeper, more restorative sleep.

>> **Avoid refined sugars, processed foods, and large amounts of carbohydrates,** which might leave you feeling groggy and less alert.

>> **Especially for children, start the day with a balanced breakfast** to improve not only sleep quality, but also motivation during morning routines.

>> **If you're a shift worker, steer clear of heavy meals during night shifts** to avoid disrupting your sleep later.

TIP

>> **Avoid alcohol and caffeine in the evening** to keep them from interfering with your ability to fall asleep or stay asleep.

Regular exercise can improve sleep quality and total sleep time (quantity). Sleep research shows that exercise can improve the symptoms and sleep quality in individuals who have sleep disorders such as insomnia, obstructive sleep apnea (OSA), restless legs syndrome (RLS), and periodic limb movements during sleep (PLMS). See Chapters 7 and 8 for more information about sleep disorders.

Recognizing Sleep Deprivation, Loss, and Disorders

Sleep deprivation is more than an occasional restless night — it's a state that affects your body, mind, and daily life. Whether caused by external factors, lifestyle habits, or underlying sleep disorders, the consequences of insufficient sleep can be profound. Recognizing the signs of sleep deprivation early is key to addressing the problem and restoring balance to your sleep-wake cycle.

REMEMBER

Avoid sleep debt — the accumulation of lost sleep over time — to prevent frequent *microsleeps.* These uncontrollable episodes of sleep can occur during the day and lead to life-threatening situations, especially when you're driving or operating hazardous machinery.

Types of sleep deprivation

Specific types of sleep deprivation can affect your sleep in various ways that curtail the amount of restful sleep you experience on a nightly basis.

>> **Acute sleep deprivation:** Not sleeping for one or more nights, either missing total or partial sleep during these nights. This may be caused, for example, by work deadlines, illness, or family situations.

>> **Chronic sleep loss and fragmentation:** Getting less sleep consistently over an extended timeframe either by a reduction in your total sleep time (voluntarily or involuntarily) or by fragmentation of your sleep.

>> **Partial and sleep-stage deprivation:** For partial sleep deprivation, your total sleep time is reduced so that you get less sleep than usual. In the case of sleep-stage deprivation, you may have a medical condition or be taking medications that reduce certain stages of sleep.

Chapter 3 guides you through recognizing and getting help for sleep deprivation.

Warning signs of sleep deprivation

Sleep deprivation can manifest in many ways, some more subtle than others:

>> **Cognitive impairments:** Difficulty concentrating, memory lapses, or slower decision-making. Sleep is essential for processing and retaining information, so even one night of poor rest can leave you feeling foggy.

>> **Emotional changes:** Increased irritability, anxiety, or mood swings. Without enough REM sleep, your brain struggles to regulate emotions effectively, and may result in or exacerbate anxiety and mood disorders, such as depression.

>> **Psychosocial changes:** Overreaction to minor annoyances, impaired social judgment, loneliness/social isolation, strained family and intimate relationships, and struggles in the workplace may be challenging effects of poor sleep.

>> **Physical symptoms:** Persistent fatigue, weakened immune function, or changes in appetite. Chronic sleep deprivation is linked to a higher risk of conditions like diabetes, heart disease, and obesity.

>> **Unintended sleep episodes:** Falling asleep during the day, even in inappropriate settings like meetings or while driving. This is a clear sign that your body is desperately trying to recover lost rest.

WARNING

If you notice any of these signs, take them seriously. Chronic sleep deprivation can have far-reaching consequences for your health and safety.

Long-term impacts of sleep loss

Prolonged sleep loss goes beyond day-to-day symptoms and increases the risk of severe health issues over time. Research shows that insufficient sleep disrupts nearly every system in the body:

>> **Cardiovascular disease:** Sleep deprivation raises blood pressure and increases inflammation, both of which contribute to heart disease and stroke.

>> **Endocrine effects:** Increased levels of cortisol and stress hormones may lead to a range of mental and physical issues.

>> **Gastrointestinal issues:** Research studies demonstrate that sleep disruption can affect the gut microbiome and lead to gastrointestinal issues such as bloating and constipation.

>> **Impaired mental health:** Chronic sleep loss is closely linked to conditions such as depression and anxiety, as well as reduced emotional resilience.

>> **Metabolic changes:** Lack of sleep disrupts the hormones that regulate hunger, leading to overeating and weight gain.

>> **Musculoskeletal effects:** Sleep loss can hamper muscle repair and growth, as well as bone density — all factors that can lead to slow recovery from injuries. And poor sleep in children can result in delayed milestones in growth patterns.

>> **Reproductive problems:** Sleep deprivation can reduce testosterone levels in men and can disrupt the menstrual cycle and affect fertility in women.

>> **Respiratory disorders:** Inadequate sleep can have an impact on preexisting respiratory conditions by exacerbating symptoms of these disorders — for example, shortness of breath and wheezing — which can contribute to even poorer sleep quality.

>> **Weakened immunity:** Your body produces infection-fighting antibodies during sleep, so poor rest leaves you more susceptible to illness.

Addressing sleep deprivation early can help reduce these risks and protect your long-term health. Chapter 6 offers strategies for improving your lifestyle to support better sleep.

Common sleep disorders

Not all sleep problems are caused by poor habits or external factors — many stem from underlying disorders that require targeted treatment. Some of the most common sleep disorders include

>> **Insomnia:** A condition in which you have difficulty falling asleep, staying asleep, or getting enough rest. This sleep disorder is one of the most common; it affects about one in six Americans. Stress, anxiety, and medical conditions are common triggers.

>> **Hypersomnias:** A group of disorders that cause symptoms such as excessive daytime sleepiness and sometimes sudden sleep attacks. Narcolepsy is a well-known hypersomnia that also features symptoms such as hallucinations when falling asleep or waking up that are frequently accompanied by temporary paralysis of voluntary muscles, and *cataplexy* (a sudden muscle weakness often triggered by strong emotions).

>> **Obstructive sleep apnea (OSA):** A common sleep-related breathing disorder that affects about 24 percent of men and 9 percent of women between the ages of 30 and 60. OSA is marked by pauses or decreases in your breathing during sleep.

>> **Restless legs syndrome (RLS):** A common condition that involves an uncontrollable urge to move the legs, especially at night, disrupting both falling asleep and staying asleep. You may also have unpleasant sensations (for example, feeling like bugs are crawling on your skin) or also experience periodic limb movements during sleep (PLMS), in which your legs kick or twitch during the night and wake you up (or, more commonly, wake up your bedpartner).

>> **Sleepwalking and sleep terrors:** Sleepwalking happens when you get up and walk around during deep sleep, even though you're not fully awake. If you've ever seen someone sleepwalking, they might seem alert, but they won't remember it the next morning. Sleep terrors, on the other hand, often happen to children. Instead of walking around, they scream or look terrified while still asleep; they are usually inconsolable and won't recall the episode the next day.

>> **Delayed sleep-wake phase disorder:** One of several circadian rhythm sleep disorders in which you struggle to fall asleep and wake up at the times you want. You might find yourself staying up late and having a hard time getting up early in the morning.

Recognizing the symptoms and signs of sleep disorders is the first step toward effective treatment. Flip to Chapters 7 and 8 for in-depth discussions of these and other sleep-related conditions.

Medical disorders and medications

Sleep disorders aren't the only causes of sleep loss. Many common medical disorders and medications — both prescription and over-the-counter (OTC) — frequently disrupt sleep. Conditions such as asthma, chronic obstructive pulmonary disease (COPD), diabetes, thyroid disease, and gastroesophageal reflux disease (GERD) can significantly impact both the quantity and quality of your sleep. Pain (physical, emotional, or psychological) is also a common cause of sleep loss.

Certain medications, including steroids, decongestants, cardiovascular drugs, and stimulants, can interfere with your ability to sleep at night. Additionally, substance abuse — particularly involving alcohol and nicotine — can severely disrupt sleep patterns. Turn to Chapter 3 to learn more about how preexisting conditions and medications can impact your sleep.

Knowing That Help Is Out There

If you've tried improving your sleep habits but continue to feel fatigued or struggle with disrupted rest, it's time to consult a professional. Sleep studies — which monitor brain activity, breathing, movement, heart rate, and blood oxygen and carbon dioxide levels — can provide valuable insights into what's happening during the night while you're sleeping (or trying to sleep). Treatment options range from behavioral therapies like cognitive behavioral therapy for insomnia (CBT-I) to medical interventions such as continuous positive airway pressure (CPAP) machines for sleep apnea.

TIP

Your primary care provider is a great place to start if you suspect a sleep disorder. They can refer you to a sleep specialist for further evaluation and treatment. Chapter 9 walks you through how to seek help for your particular concerns.

Struggling with sleep can feel isolating, but it's important to remember that you're not alone — and solutions are within reach. Sleep issues are incredibly common, affecting millions of people worldwide, and the good news is that there are effective treatments and resources available to help you reclaim restful nights.

Managing your sleep

To help improve your sleep, you can try

>> **Improving sleep hygiene/habits:** These habits include maintaining a consistent sleep-wake schedule, creating a comfortable bedroom

environment, managing light resources, establishing a sleep-supporting pre-bedtime behavior pattern, and avoiding staying in bed longer than 20 minutes if you can't fall asleep or fall back to sleep.

>> **Using medications:** Prescription or OTC medications are rarely a long-term answer to improving your sleep or daytime sleepiness, but they can be helpful in breaking the cycle of poor sleep before it becomes a chronic condition. In this context, medications such as melatonin may be beneficial under the supervision of a physician.

>> **Short-term countermeasures for occasional sleep loss:** Brief naps (10–20 minutes) can help improve your alertness without resulting in grogginess. Caffeine can also temporarily boost your alertness.

Visit Chapters 3, 6, and 15 for much more on how to maintain high-quality sleep.

Getting help from a sleep specialist

When you see a sleep specialist, they not only discuss your sleep problems, medical history, and daily habits with you, but also conduct a physical examination. The physician focuses on evaluating your sleep issues to decide on whether you need a sleep study or other specialized tests such as

>> **Actigraphy:** A method to monitor human rest and activity cycles by using a device (actigraph) that usually resembles a wristwatch and records movement through an accelerometer. The actigraphy data can provide information regarding sleep patterns and sleep-wake cycles of activity over extended periods, which is most helpful for circadian rhythm issues.

>> **Home sleep tests (HSTs):** Tests that typically help diagnose obstructive sleep apnea, and directly or indirectly measure your airflow, breathing effort, blood oxygen levels, heart rate, and body position.

>> **Maintenance of Wakefulness Test (MWT):** A daytime test that measures your ability to stay awake when seated in a semi-darkened room. This test includes four 40-minute trials — each spaced two hours apart. The goal is to demonstrate your ability to stay awake for the duration of the 40-minute trials, without environmental stimulation. This test has helped commercial drivers and pilots to return to duty after successful treatment.

>> **Multiple Sleep Latency Test (MSLT):** A daytime test consisting of a series of up to five scheduled naps designed to evaluate your propensity to fall asleep. If you need to take this test, it generally happens immediately following a night spent in a sleep lab to add upon the data produced during that overnight sleep test.

>> **Polysomnography (PSG):** A daytime or nighttime in-laboratory sleep study to measure the way your body functions during sleep. The data obtained is comprehensive and runs the gamut from measuring sleep efficiency (time spent asleep versus time in bed) to body positions, sleep stages, and abnormal breathing events.

To discover more about these sleep tests, turn to Chapter 10.

Exploring treatment options

Sleep problems vary widely, so the treatment you receive depends on your specific issue. If you see your doctor or a sleep specialist, they may recommend one or more common approaches:

>> **Behavioral therapies:** Cognitive behavioral therapy for insomnia (CBT-I) is a gold-standard treatment for those struggling to fall or stay asleep or change their sleep schedule. This therapy helps you identify and eliminate unhelpful thought patterns and behaviors that disrupt sleep. See Chapter 7 for more on managing insomnia and how CBT-I works.

>> **Lifestyle adjustments:** Improving your sleep hygiene (habits) — such as sticking to a regular sleep schedule, creating a calming bedtime routine and environment, and limiting caffeine intake — can make a significant difference for many people. Chapter 6 delves into actionable strategies for adopting healthier sleep habits, and Chapter 3 offers tips for setting up a sleep-friendly environment.

>> **Medical interventions:** Conditions such as sleep apnea or narcolepsy often require medical treatment. Continuous positive airway pressure (CPAP) machines, for example, are highly effective for managing sleep apnea and medications (stimulants or suppressants) may help with other disorders such as narcolepsy or restless legs syndrome. Chapters 7 and 8 have more information about medical interventions for specific sleep disorders.

REMEMBER

Don't hesitate to seek help for a sleep disorder. Whether your treatment involves therapy, medication, or a combination of approaches, you can find proven solutions to address even the most stubborn sleep challenges.

Finding resources for support

The process of improving your sleep might take time, but even small steps can lead to noticeable changes. Whether you incorporate relaxation techniques in your bedtime routine, adjust your sleep schedule, or seek professional help, every effort brings you closer to the rest you deserve. And navigating sleep challenges doesn't have to be a solo journey. Many resources are available to guide you toward better sleep:

>> **Educational tools:** Books (like this one!) and reputable online resources, such as the American Academy of Sleep Medicine (AASM) at https://sleepeducation.org or the National Sleep Foundation at www.thensf.org, can empower you with knowledge and strategies to improve your sleep.

>> **Sleep specialists and clinics:** Accredited sleep centers offer diagnostic tests, like *polysomnography* (PSG, sleep studies), to pinpoint specific disorders. These tests monitor brain activity, breathing, and muscle movements to provide a comprehensive picture of important changes in your body during sleep. Learn more about what to expect during a sleep study in Chapter 10.

>> **Support groups:** Connecting with others who face similar sleep challenges can provide emotional support and practical tips. Online forums, local meetups, and patient advocacy organizations are great places to start.

TIP

If you're unsure where to start, ask your primary care provider for a referral to a sleep specialist for further evaluation and treatment. They can help you navigate the options and determine the best path forward. Chapter 9 walks you through how to seek help for your particular concerns.

IN THIS CHAPTER

» **Investigating brain waves while you're awake and asleep**

» **Sifting through the states and stages**

» **Diving into the history of sleep discoveries**

» **Uncovering sleep habits in the animal kingdom**

Chapter **2**

Delving Into the Science of Sleep

S cientists have studied sleep for centuries, uncovering its complexities and importance. You might already know that sleep is divided into stages, but did you know these stages each have unique identifying features? From light sleep to deep sleep — and the intriguing world of rapid eye movement (REM) and non-REM states of sleep — each stage (with its features) is a piece of the puzzle that makes up a good (or not so good) night's rest. And scientists know humans aren't the only species who experience these sleep stages; many animals share similar sleep patterns.

But how and why does this sleep process work? In this chapter, I take you through the universal need for sleep across species, the science of how your brain and other body parts work together to generate and benefit from sleep, and how people have come to understand sleep so well.

Although sleep explorers have so much more to learn, thanks to ongoing research and remarkable discoveries throughout the 20th century, scientists know more than ever about how sleep affects your memory, mood, and overall well-being. Diving into the science of sleep allows you to appreciate why it is so crucial and how it impacts every aspect of your life.

Understanding Wakefulness

To understand sleep states and stages, you first have to understand what happens when you're awake. When you're awake, your brain is in an active state in which it processes information and controls your body's movements (among other things). Your brain receives input from your eyes, ears, skin, and other senses and integrates this information to help you navigate and respond to your surroundings. It also coordinates your thoughts, emotions, and voluntary actions, enabling you to perform tasks, communicate, and engage with the world.

When you're awake, your brain waves are primarily *alpha* and *beta* waves. Sleep specialists can see these waves by using sleep lab equipment called *polysomnography* (PSG), which measures electrical activity in your brain, eyes, muscles, and heart, and also assesses breathing parameters. When sleep specialists determine your states and stages of sleep, they look at three main types of PSG:

>> **Electroencephalography (EEG),** which measures your brain waves

>> **Electrooculography (EOG),** which measures your eye movements

>> **Electromyography (EMG),** which measures the movements of other muscles, like your chin

You can read in-depth about the different types of PSG and how they work in Chapter 10.

Brain waves incorporate various forms and frequencies depending on your state of wakefulness (versus sleep) and your level of activity. They include

>> **Alpha waves,** which occur when you close your eyes while you're still awake but relaxed and not actively processing much information — maybe when you're meditating or just resting your eyes for a moment. These waves are uniform and rhythmic and have a frequency of 8 to 13 cycles per second (measured in hertz or Hz).

>> **Beta waves** that are present when you're actively engaged in mental activities, such as problem-solving, critical thinking, or decision-making. Beta waves have a frequency of 13 Hz or higher, and they indicate an alert and focused mind. Actually, a mixed frequency pattern of alpha, beta, and even *theta* waves occurs when your eyes are open. Additionally, your EOG and EMG show mixed patterns reflecting movement of the muscles while you're awake.

>> **Theta waves,** which become more apparent as you start to transition away from wakefulness to sleep. You get drowsy or tired, your body's movements decrease, and your brain waves slow down to a lower frequency in the range of 4 to 8 Hz.

Figure 2-1 shows how your various brain waves look in wakefulness and drowsiness when monitored by PSG.

Some Brain Waves Measured in a Sleep Lab

Wave Type	Frequency Range	Waveform	Happens When You Are
Alpha	8–13 Hz		Relaxing with eyes closed
Beta	13–30 Hz		Actively engaging in mental activities
Theta	4–8 Hz		During drowsiness and stages N1 and N2 (light sleep)

FIGURE 2-1: Alpha, beta, and theta waves.

A Tale of Two States of Sleep: REM and non-REM (NREM)

There are two states of sleep: REM (rapid eye movement) and non-REM (NREM) sleep. Sleep specialists use these two broad terms for sleep states, and add subdivisions that they call sleep stages (although REM sleep is sometimes also referred to as a stage of sleep).

Recognizing REM

REM sleep typically occurs about 90 to 120 minutes after you fall asleep and recurs multiple times throughout the night, with each REM period getting longer.

REMEMBER

A person who has the sleep disorder narcolepsy can have sleep-onset REM periods, meaning that they can transition very quickly from wakefulness to light sleep and to REM sleep in 15–20 minutes instead of the usual 90–120 minutes.

Scientists believe this state is essential for emotional regulation, memory consolidation, and brain development. REM sleep periods have these characteristics:

>> **Cardiorespiratory instability,** a condition in which your heart rate can become irregular, and your breathing can become shallow and also irregular.

>> **Brain activity that is similar to the brain activity when you're awake,** but your body becomes relaxed and still. About 90 percent of your dreams happen during REM sleep, and your eyes move around quickly in different directions during this state (often correlating to what you're dreaming about), but they don't send visual information to your sleeping brain.

>> **Muscle paralysis,** that is, the majority of your voluntary muscles become completely paralyzed.

REMEMBER

Not all muscles are paralyzed during REM sleep. The involuntary muscles that are necessary to sustain life (for example, the heart and muscles needed for breathing) remain unaffected, as do your eye muscles and — interestingly — the muscles in your middle ear.

Sleep specialists consider REM sleep both a state and a stage of sleep. They sometimes label it as a *state* of sleep because it is a condition of the brain/mind during sleep (NREM and REM), but they also sometimes label it as a *stage* of sleep along with the subdivisions of NREM (N1, N2, N3, REM).

Identifying NREM

NREM sleep is the foundation of your restorative sleep. During NREM sleep, scientists believe that your body undergoes essential repair processes, such as tissue growth and muscle recovery, while your brain perhaps consolidates memories and clears out metabolic waste. During this state, your brain waves are slower and your physiological activity decreases, maybe allowing your body and mind to rejuvenate. NREM sleep makes up the majority of your sleep cycle, providing the deep rest necessary for overall well-being.

Sleep scientists subdivide NREM into three stages: N1, N2, N3. To identify which stage of sleep you're in, your specialist typically looks at three indicators during a sleep study:

>> **Your brain waves.** Specialists look at your *electroencephalography* (EEG) or brain waves in 30-second intervals called *epochs*. Your sleep specialist deems you to be in a certain sleep stage if your brain waves remain in one stage for more than 15 seconds of one epoch.

>> **Your eye movements.** Using *electrooculography* (EOG), your specialist measures how fast or slow your eyes move while you're sleeping. To read about how the electrical charges in your eyes work, see the sidebar "More about measuring eye movements," and to read about EOG technology, turn to Chapter 10.

>> **Your chin muscle movements.** Using chin *electromyography* (EMG), your specialist monitors for a decrease in muscle tension as you fall asleep. Flip to Chapter 10 to read about the technology behind EMG.

Stage N1: Light sleep

Stage N1 sleep is the lightest and often first stage of NREM sleep. During N1 sleep, your brain waves are predominantly theta waves. Stage N1 sleep also features slow, rolling eye movements and relaxed chin muscles.

N1 sleep is such a light sleep that sometimes, people don't even realize they are sleeping when they are in this stage. For example, as part of sleep-related research, we sleep specialists may wake patients up throughout different stages of sleep to evaluate them, and if I wake a patient up after several epochs of N1 sleep and ask them what they remember about their sleep, I often get a response like "Why are you disturbing me? I wasn't sleeping yet!"

Another common example that you might recognize from your own life is that moment when, say, you're driving, and all of a sudden, you feel yourself jolt awake, even though you didn't know you were sleeping. That's N1 sleep — or what sleep specialists call a *microsleep* (a sudden temporary episode of sleep that lasts for a few seconds).

WARNING

N1 sleep can occur suddenly, and the person is usually *amnestic* (not aware of it).

In addition to the suddenness of the onset of sleep and the accompanying amnesia, some behavioral events can occur at the beginning of sleep. You may experience any of the following:

>> **A hypnic jerk or *sleep start*,** which is characterized by a full-body twitch or jerk that is often accompanied by a sensation of falling. This is a benign phenomenon and is thought to occur because of a temporary interruption of a descending wave of inhibition of muscle activity from the brain to the nerves and muscles of the body.

>> **Recall of fragmentary images** that occurs if you wake up after falling sleep. You might recall brief images that you experienced before falling asleep (for example, your bedpartner's face or the page of a book you were reading).

>> **Automatic behavior** that manifests as unrecognizable scribbles in your notebook — indicating that you might have fallen asleep while writing (this often happens to sleep-deprived students as they struggle to remain awake during lectures!) — or speaking unintelligible words during a phone conversation while drowsy.

Stage N2: Intermediate sleep

N2 sleep is the most common sleep stage, comprising 40 to 55 percent of your nightly sleep. During N2 sleep, your body begins to relax more significantly: Your heart rate slows down, your body temperature drops, and your muscles become less tense. Brain activity also slows, but it includes brief bursts of rapid brain waves known as *sleep spindles* and sudden peaks called *K-complexes*. Sleep specialists believe that these unique patterns help your brain process and consolidate memories, as well as suppress external stimuli so that you can sleep well. The features of sleep spindles and K-complexes (depicted in Figure 2-2) are interesting:

>> **Sleep spindles** are EEG patterns that start off small, get higher in frequency (12–14 cycles per second), and then get small again after half a second or more, making this waveform resemble a yarn spindle.

>> **K-complexes (KC)** are brain wave patterns on an EEG that show a sharp negative wave followed by a positive wave that stands out from the background EEG for half a second or more. **Note:** Negative is up and positive is down in EEGs. K-complexes usually appear on the sleep study generated by the central electrode, which is the electrode that goes along the central line (called a sulcus) of your brain.

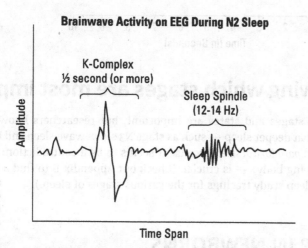

Brainwave Activity on EEG During N2 Sleep

K-Complex
½ second (or more)

Sleep Spindle
(12-14 Hz)

Amplitude

Time Span

FIGURE 2-2: How sleep spindles and K-complexes look in EEGs.

REMEMBER

There are no specific amplitude criteria for either K-complexes or sleep spindles.

In the sleep lab, when sleep specialists wake patients up from N2 sleep, they typically remember that they were sleeping.

Stage N3: Deepest sleep

N3 sleep is also called *slow wave sleep* or *deep sleep*. This is the deepest and most restorative stage of NREM sleep. Two hallmarks of N3 sleep on an EEG — see Figure 2-3 — illustrate that your brain waves

>> Are *delta* waves that have a frequency of .5-4 Hz

>> Show an amplitude (or height) of over 75 microvolts

This N3 stage is critical for physical recovery, as your body focuses on repairing tissues, building bone and muscle, and strengthening the immune system. N3 sleep also plays a significant role in consolidating long-term memories and clearing out toxins from the brain. But here's a catch: Because it is the most rejuvenating stage, waking up in the middle of N3 sleep can leave you feeling groggy and disoriented, a phenomenon known as *sleep inertia*.

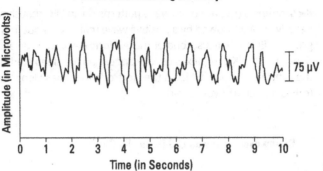

Delta Waves During N3 Sleep

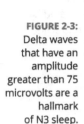

FIGURE 2-3:
Delta waves that have an amplitude greater than 75 microvolts are a hallmark of N3 sleep.

Knowing which stages are most important

All sleep stages and states are important, but researchers know from years of studies that deeper sleep — such as stage N3 slow-wave sleep and REM sleep (also known as *paradoxical sleep* because it seems to be a contradiction: an active brain in a sleeping body) — is crucial. (Check out Appendix B to find a series of actual human sleep study tracings for the various stages of sleep.)

SLEEP IN NEWBORNS

Newborns experience three sleep stages that are different from those of older people: quiet sleep, active sleep, and indeterminate sleep.

- **Quiet sleep** is analogous to NREM sleep, and has a discontinuous EEG pattern in which intermittent electrical activity bursts alternate with quiet periods. The EMG activity may be low with a few body movements, and the heart rate and breathing are regular.

- **Active sleep** is present after 32 weeks' gestation, and is analogous to REM sleep with a characteristic REM EEG, rapid eye movements, a variable EMG with frequent body movements, grimaces, and twitches, and a variable heart and breathing rate.

- **Indeterminate sleep** means that specialists can't distinguish quiet from active sleep in the sleep study.

As a newborn ages, the EEG rhythm detected in the occipital regions (back of the head) in relaxed wakefulness with the eyes closed gradually increases in frequency from 3.5 to 4.5 Hz at 3 to 4 months, to 6 Hz at 12 months, and then to the normal alpha frequency at 8 years of age.

Studies on rats deprived of N3 and paradoxical sleep show that they typically die at an average of 10 to 15 days if deprived of total sleep, and they generally die at an average of 27 days if deprived of paradoxical sleep.

Researchers don't entirely know why certain situations happen, but their findings also include these:

>> **Increased infection rates:** Despite the fact that the rats' immune function seems to remain intact, many rats studied contract infections and die near the end of the sleep deprivation period.

>> **Increased metabolic rates:** The rats' metabolic rate tends to increase, meaning they eat more, but still lose body weight.

>> **Decreased body temperature:** Within the 72 hours before they die, rats experience a rapid decrease in body temperature. This suggests that sleep deprivation affects metabolism, regardless of the sleep state.

Although researchers conduct these studies on animals, sleep specialists can take clues from them for insights about humans. Limited studies of sleep deprivation in young, healthy adults in the 1950s–1960s have shown that their metabolism seems to slightly increase, as they tend to eat more and lose some body weight. We know that the deeper stages of sleep and paradoxical sleep are particularly important, whereas lighter stages of sleep deprivation do not seem to have as profound an effect.

TECHNICAL
STUFF

Just because depriving an animal or human of sleep causes certain adverse conditions to occur, this does not necessarily mean that these conditions are the sole function of sleep. For example, sleep loss might affect metabolism and temperature regulation, but this doesn't conclusively explain why sleep is necessary. Also, although N3 and paradoxical (REM) sleep appear to be more important, researchers don't conclusively know why.

Looking at Early Investigations into Sleep and Sleep Deprivation

Some of the earliest researchers who published their findings on sleep were

>> **Marie de Manacéïne,** who published a book in 1897 (the early days of sleep research) entitled *Sleep: Its Physiology, Pathology, Hygiene and Psychology.*

This book involved sleep deprivation studies on animals. Manacéïne found that the sleep-deprived animals uniformly decreased their body temperature, had decreased numbers of red and white blood cells, and died after a few days of sleep deprivation. Her book also describes sleep disorders such as insomnia, narcolepsy, and sleepwalking, and discusses the study and significance of dreams. At the time, her book was considered a comprehensive work on sleep, with many countries distributing it.

>> **Henri Piéron,** who published his seminal book, *Le Problème Physiologique du Sommeil (The Physiological Problem of Sleep)*, in 1913.

In his book, Piéron proposed different theories of sleep without being totally conclusive. But one of his greatest contributions was that he noted changes in respiration, digestive secretions (like sweat, tears, and urine), temperature, and other systems. He put forth the *toxin theory*, suggesting that without sleep, toxins build up and cause bodily harm.

>> **Nathaniel Kleitman,** who is considered to be "the grandfather of sleep research," published *Sleep and Wakefulness* in 1939.

Kleitman's book, revised in 1963, covers the disorders that researchers knew about at the time, including narcolepsy, insomnia, and other sleep disturbances. It also reviews topics such as hibernation, hypnosis, and attempts to control or modify sleep. This book and Kleitman's pioneering research led to his peers giving him the "grandfather" nickname.

SLEEP IN EARLIER TIMES

Sleep researchers have gathered the most information about sleep in earlier times by looking at some of the bed surfaces and objects such as pillows, which were less comfortable than those we have today. Even in ancient Egyptian times, people used a type of rigid headrest that would actually elevate their heads and necks. Some cultures still sleep on relatively hard surfaces in modern times.

Dr. Jerome Siegel of UCLA studied the sleep patterns of three Indigenous societies — the Hadza of Tanzania, the San of Namibia, and the Tsimané of Bolivia — to explore what sleep might have been like in early humans. He found that these groups averaged six and a half hours of sleep per night, debunking the myth that people slept from sunset to sunrise. They stayed up about three hours past dusk and woke up when the temperature reached its lowest point during the night. This suggests that our sleep patterns may not be so different from those of early humans, despite modern technology.

Medieval literature and pre-industrial accounts mention the concept of *biphasic sleep*, in which people initially slept from about 9 p.m. to 11 p.m. They would then awaken and do household chores, work, socialize, or conduct other activities for a few hours; then they slept again, usually until dawn. Following the advent of electric lights, biphasic sleep has largely disappeared in modern culture. However, in limited research conducted in light-deprived environments, biphasic sleep patterns have been shown to emerge after a few weeks in this condition.

Interestingly, younger individuals in today's world can sleep in almost any environment because they can sleep more deeply and efficiently than older people. But as people age, bed comfort becomes more important due to less efficient sleep and more frequent interruptions from medical and sleep conditions. And so, modern bed technology comes in very handy. Today, people can buy various types of mattresses and pillows that have different composition and firmness, and even technology that allows them to adjust positions and firmness during sleep.

Applauding the Discovery of REM Sleep

In September 1953, graduate student Eugene Aserinsky and his dissertation advisor, Dr. Nathaniel Kleitman, reported their discovery of REM sleep while using PSG at the University of Chicago in a brief article published in the journal *Science*, entitled "Regularly Occurring Periods of Eye Motility, and Concomitant Phenomena, During Sleep." As Aserinsky studied individuals sleeping, he noticed periods during sleep when the patients' eyes moved rapidly under their eyelids, which they subsequently called rapid eye movement sleep. Aserinsky later noted that these REM periods often correlated with dream recall when he awakened individuals from REM.

Their discovery was pivotal in the scientific study of sleep. Before it, researchers hadn't reported different components of sleep in their scientific literature. After Aserinsky and Kleitman discovered REM sleep, more researchers started exploring sleep in depth. Regarding dreaming, they found that

» **Most dreaming occurs during REM sleep.**

» **Dreaming is often continuous,** meaning that when people wake up during REM sleep and then go back to sleep, they often continue the dreams they were having. This is much like reading different chapters of the same book.

DR. DEMENT AND HIS DEARTH OF DREAMS

One funny anecdote about dreaming and REM sleep comes from Dr. William Dement, considered "the father of sleep medicine." He often recounted a story — which he also shares in his 1999 book, *The Promise of Sleep* — about how he became so interested in REM sleep that he volunteered as a research subject. He had done so many studies on other people where he woke up his patients during REM sleep and they would recount their dreams in such vivid detail that he wanted to experience this as well.

Dr. Dement trained a research assistant to wake him up during REM sleep, but much to his chagrin, he couldn't recall any dreams, and he became very distressed and confused. After a few nights of this situation, he became very embarrassed and worried. What if he ended up being the first person who didn't have dreams while in REM sleep? And he almost made up dreams to share.

As it turned out, he apparently hadn't trained the research assistant well, because the assistant was waking Dr. Dement during a different stage of sleep! The silver lining is that his experience did corroborate his theory that 90 percent of dreams occur during REM sleep.

REMEMBER

This discovery of REM sleep launched the sleep research field into further studies. Psychiatrists and psychologists took a special interest soon after REM's discovery because they believed that studying dream content during REM sleep could possibly provide them with insights into the mind and mental illnesses.

Examining Sleep in Other Species

Researchers know that sleep varies *phylogenetically*, meaning that differences across species exist, and similarities between species can be evolutionarily linked. In general, sleep habits — including the places where animals sleep and the postures they take while sleeping — vary widely.

Interestingly, one of my first projects as a graduate student involved spending many hours with a microscope looking at paramecium to identify any behavior that simulated sleep. I did observe that they had what appeared to be a basic rest cycle where they stopped moving, and then other cycles where they were more active. Whether or not those cycles illustrate actual sleep or a surrogate for sleep is inconclusive.

In order for researchers to study sleep in other species, they have to able to record sleep (including their brain activity and sometimes muscle activity) using EEG and EMG, respectively. This is simply impossible for some species, so researchers don't know everything about how every species sleeps. Particularly mysterious are single-cell organisms like bacteria. These organisms have periods where they rest or stop activity, but scientists don't know whether it qualifies as sleep because they cannot yet measure it properly.

Evaluating sleep in nonhumans

For insects, behavioral criteria define what constitutes sleep, and researchers find stereotypic postures that are species-specific for sleeping insects. In particular, scientists have studied sleep and circadian rhythms in cockroaches, mosquitos, honeybees, and fruit flies.

Through pioneering work on fruit flies (*Drosophila melanogaster*), Drs. Jeffrey Hall, Michael Rosbash, and Michael Young isolated and characterized a gene that comprises the clock that governs circadian rhythms. This pioneering work led to the trio sharing the Nobel Prize in Physiology or Medicine in 2017.

Sleep research focused on other species has yielded mixed results. Although debatable, components of REM and NREM sleep might exist in reptiles, and studies of amphibians using electrodes to assess brain, eye, and muscle activity have shown contradictory results for determining the presence of different sleep states. However, even to this day, researchers don't know whether these species have alternating cycles or true states of sleep.

Sleeping with half a brain

A particularly interesting phenomenon, *unihemispheric sleep*, occurs in some aquatic species, such as cetaceans (whales, dolphins, and porpoises). These species sleep with only one hemisphere of their brain at a time so that they can still swim. And it's unclear whether or not cetaceans have REM sleep. Researchers have also observed unihemispheric sleep in birds, noting that birds often keep one eye open during NREM sleep.

Interestingly, a version of this phenomenon can occur in humans as well. It's not that one hemisphere can be totally asleep while the other is awake; rather, as a result of strokes or tumors, one hemisphere of the brain may be in a different stage or state of sleep than the other. I personally saw this condition many years ago in a patient who had a ruptured blood vessel in her brainstem that resulted in showing the characteristic EEG pattern of REM sleep in one hemisphere of her brain but not the other. This patient also had typical rapid eye movements and decreased muscle activity during REM sleep.

DO SHARKS SLEEP?

Researchers don't currently know whether sharks sleep, have unihemispheric sleep, or sleep facing ocean currents that allow the oxygenated water to pass through their gills and allow them to rest while still getting the oxygen they need. Scientists think that sharks must swim to breathe, but researchers have observed sharks having behavioral rest periods.

Some sharks are called *obligate ram ventilators*, meaning that they pull oxygen-rich sea water through their mouths and force it out of their gills while swimming. Other species, called *buccal pumpers*, pull water in through their mouths and force it out through the gills by their cheek muscles. And other types of sharks are able to remain stationary while forcing water through their gills by using specialized structures called *spiracles*.

Noting sleep similarities between animals

Researchers also know that mammals sleep and most likely all experience cyclical alternation between REM and NREM sleep. *Note:* One notable exception is the *spiny anteater* (or *echidna*), which may have REM sleep only in certain conditions, such as being at the right temperature.

Birds and mammals exhibit sleep states that are similar, but also have some differences. For example, scientists find

>> Some EEG rhythms in mammals but not in birds, and although birds have reduced muscle activity in REM sleep, it's not to the same degree as in mammals.

>> That, although birds do have alternating REM and NREM sleep, the cycles are very short. This situation makes sense, given their need to maintain balance while perching or flying. Birds can also exhibit behavior that looks like *power naps* (short sleep taken during a working day), where their eyes are partially closed and feathers are fluffed for a few seconds to a few minutes before they become more alert and awake again.

Within the sleep medicine research community, people think that birds and mammals developed REM sleep independently of each other because birds are classified as a type of reptile and last shared a common ancestor with mammals over 300 million years ago.

TIP

To keep all of the species' sleep habits straight, you can remember that a loose association exists between body mass and the typical amount of sleep over a 24-hour period. Larger animals — such as giraffes and elephants — tend to sleep less (typically less than 5 hours), while smaller animals such as bats sleep much longer (around 19 or 20 hours). Humans and household pets such as cats fall in between, clocking in at around 7 hours and 12 hours, respectively.

Searching for the Holy Grail: Why We Sleep

Former University of Chicago professor Dr. Allan Rechtschaffen, who was one of my mentors and a pioneer in the field of sleep medicine, said

> "If sleep does not serve an absolutely vital function, then it is the biggest mistake the evolutionary process ever made."

Dr. Rechtschaffen dedicated his life to the pursuit of discovering the overall function of sleep, which is considered the Holy Grail of the sleep field. But despite his best efforts and those of his team, the question of why humans and animals sleep remains unanswered.

Early theories

Throughout history, scholars and philosophers have speculated about the purpose and causes of sleep. Here are some of the key early theories:

>> **Substance accumulation hypothesis:** An early idea proposed that an unknown substance that causes fatigue accumulated in the body during wakefulness and dissipated during sleep to restore alertness.

>> **Philosophical perspective:** Philosophers, including Plato, speculated that sleep could create a division between the body and soul, possibly allowing for a separation or a different state of consciousness.

>> **Aristotle's vapor theory:** Aristotle believed that sleep resulted from warm vapors rising from the stomach, which explained the tendency to feel drowsy after eating.

>> **Cerebral anemia theory:** Later medical theories suggested that sleep was caused by *cerebral anemia*, a situation in which blood flow was diverted away from the brain to other parts of the body, particularly the gut.

>> **Lack of environmental stimulation:** Another hypothesis posited that sleep occurs when a lack of environmental stimuli occurs, leading to a natural tendency to drift into sleep when nothing engaging is happening.

These theories, while now outdated, laid the groundwork for our modern understanding of sleep and its complexities.

Prevailing theories

One current key theory is that sleep is necessary for restoration and recovery, helping to reverse and restore biological, biochemical, and physiological processes that degrade during wakefulness. However, decreased protein synthesis occurs during sleep, so this theory doesn't explain everything. But in 2013, experiments on mice showed a 60 percent increase in the clearance of waste products, such as beta-amyloid, from the brain during sleep. This suggests that people sleep to remove potentially neurotoxic waste products that accumulate in the central nervous system during wakefulness.

TIP

Researchers have linked Alzheimer's in humans to a buildup of beta-amyloid, strengthening the argument that getting proper sleep can help lower your risk for getting the disease.

Another theory is energy conservation, proposing that sleep helps preserve energy. However, the metabolic rate during sleep reduces only by about 15 percent, which seems insufficient to explain the natural selection of sleep for preserving energy since this reduction seems minor given the prolonged period (around 8 hours) of physical activity. The calorie savings from eight hours of sleep are only about 120 calories.

During my graduate days, I helped Dr. Rechtschaffen conduct pivotal experiments into sleep deprivation. We found that when rats were deprived of sleep, they increased their metabolic rate (for example, they ate almost two and a half times more than their regular amount of food) but still lost weight. This phenomenon occurred regardless of the sleep stage of which they were deprived. And so, the research team led by Dr. Rechtschaffen thought that maybe the increase in metabolism was a result of their drop in body temperature during the course of sleep deprivation, which suggests that thermoregulation and metabolism might be functions of sleep. But to be honest, the jury is still out.

A few more theories

Despite the intense study of sleep since the early 1950s, the exact function of sleep remains a biological enigma. Still, although scientists don't necessarily know why humans and animals sleep, they have identified some of the critical brain structures involved in sleep and circadian rhythms, the neurotransmitters that drive or are associated with sleep, and some of the central nervous system pathways that are responsible for initiating and maintaining the different sleep stages. (Turn to Chapter 4 for the detailed explanation of the connection between sleep and circadian rhythms.)

Research has proposed another couple of theories to tackle the sleep enigma:

>> **An ecological hypothesis** suggests that sleep may decrease animals' vulnerability to predators by reducing their activity and chances of being spotted. However, simply resting could achieve the same effect.

>> **Other theories address organizational reasons for sleep,** such as preserving neural pathways for eye movements, reverse learning to purge unimportant information, general homeostasis (preserving a stable equilibrium of physiological processes), and memory consolidation, where sleep helps convert short-term memories into long-term storage.

REMEMBER

Overall, sleep researchers know that REM sleep deprivation during critical developmental periods can produce long-lasting changes in brain function and nearly every organ system. However, while these deprivation studies show effects, they don't necessarily explain the function of sleep. If you remove something such as sleep and observe an effect, this doesn't necessarily mean that the thing that was removed was responsible for the effect.

THE DANGERS OF TOO LITTLE OR TOO MUCH SLEEP

You probably already know that getting too little sleep can negatively impact your health, but did you know that getting too much can do the same? Sleep researchers have discovered a U-shaped survival curve: People who regularly get less than four hours or more than ten hours of sleep per night tend to have increased mortality. Studies have included controls for various factors, such as tobacco intake, body weight, medications, and other medical conditions, and found that sleep is still the determining factor.

An average adult typically needs about seven hours of sleep per night. Getting anything less often can result in physiological and other consequences (turn to Chapter 3 for more on these). You know you're getting too little sleep if you often feel or look tired during the day or want to take a lot of breaks or naps throughout your day. You might also experience microsleeps, whether or not you're aware of them. People getting too little sleep may also feel irritable or unable to manage their moods well.

On the opposite side, despite social media trends (for example, TikTok *sleepmaxxing*, which centers on improving sleep quality and quantity by exploring, and obsessing over, various products, techniques, and strategies for achieving more restorative rest), getting more than nine to ten hours of sleep nightly can also cause problems.

(continued)

(continued)

Studies have shown that individuals who get too much sleep may have

- A higher risk of medical disorders such as heart disease, diabetes, and obesity (however, whether the excess sleep is associated with or caused by these medical disorders is unclear).

- Links to mental health problems such as depression.

- Potential underlying health problems, such as sleep disorders or other medical conditions (turn to Chapters 7 and 8 to read all about sleep disorders).

If you get too little or too much sleep — and notice that this situation has an impact on your daily life — seeing a specialist is important.

IN THIS CHAPTER

» Surveying the basics of sleep deprivation

» Uncovering the causes of sleep loss

» Exploring the impact of sleep deprivation on body systems

» Seeing what sleep loss does to your behavior

» Treating sleep loss and deprivation

Chapter **3**

Evaluating Inadequate Sleep: Deprivation and Loss

Despite the importance of sleep, many people struggle to get enough rest, leading to a host of physical, mental, and emotional challenges. In our fast-paced world, sleep often takes a backseat to work, social obligations, and personal interests. However, understanding the significance of sleep and the consequences of deprivation can empower you to make better choices for adopting healthy sleep habits that positively impact your overall health. This chapter delves into the complexities of sleep deprivation, shedding light on why it happens and how it affects every facet of your life.

By the way, although I use the terms sleep deprivation and sleep loss interchangeably in this chapter, *sleep loss* is a broad term that means any decrease in the amount of sleep, whereas *sleep deprivation* is usually considered a type of sleep loss that is self-imposed or due to extrinsic factors that aren't completely under your control. For example, you may be subject to stressful work or family responsibilities, or you may be participating in sleep research experiments in which your sleep is directly or indirectly reduced.

Sleep is more than just a passive state; it's a critical component of your overall health and well-being. From understanding the mechanics of sleep debt to exploring the consequences of inadequate rest, this chapter helps you uncover the reasons why getting enough quality sleep is essential. You also learn about the various factors that contribute to sleep loss, including environmental influences, medical conditions, and lifestyle choices. By recognizing these factors, you can take proactive steps to improve your sleep hygiene and mitigate the adverse effects of sleep deprivation.

Whether you're a busy professional, a parent, or someone struggling with insomnia, the insights and strategies in this chapter help you navigate the challenges of sleep deprivation.

Understanding the Nuts and Bolts of Sleep Deprivation

Sleep deprivation isn't just about feeling tired; it encompasses a range of conditions that can significantly impact your physical and mental well-being. This section dives into the essential concepts of sleep debt, acute and partial sleep deprivation, and chronic sleep loss. Different types of sleep deprivation affect your body and mind, and understanding these distinctions is crucial for identifying whether you have sleep deprivation and what you can do to combat it. Whether you're missing a few hours of sleep here and there or consistently not getting enough rest, the consequences can be profound. Here are the nuts and bolts of what happens when you don't get enough sleep.

The concepts of sleep debt and sleep satiation

Sleep debt is like a credit card balance that grows when you don't get enough sleep. Each time you fall short of your necessary sleep, you're essentially borrowing hours. This debt accumulates over time, leading to more significant deficits in alertness and overall well-being. Just like financial debt, sleep debt can become unmanageable if you don't address it. The result of ignoring sleep debt can include frequent, irresistible, and uncontrollable episodes of sleep, known as *microsleeps*, during the day.

WARNING

Microsleeps can happen at the most inconvenient times, such as during work or while driving, severely impacting your daily functioning and even threatening your life if you are behind the wheel.

On the flip side, *sleep satiation* refers to the process of indulging in extra sleep, often over 10 hours in bed, to recover from sleep debt. While this indulgence might seem like a luxury, studies suggest that extended sleep doesn't necessarily boost alertness beyond a certain point. It can help pay back some of the lost sleep, but it's not always a one-to-one recovery.

REMEMBER

If you lose three hours of sleep, a single good night's sleep with an added three hours of sleep may not completely compensate for the effects of the lost hours. As Figure 3-1 depicts, acquiring sleep debt is a gradual process, and sleep satiation can aid in mitigating the effects of accumulated sleep debt by improving your mood, cognitive functions, and overall health.

The Progression of Sleep Debt

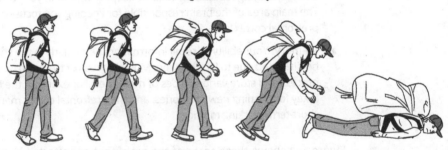

FIGURE 3-1:
Sleep debt doesn't disappear until you pay it back.

Acute sleep deprivation

Acute sleep deprivation happens when you skip sleep for one or more nights. This period of skipping sleep can involve either total sleep loss or partial sleep loss, where you get some sleep but less than your usual amount. This scenario can happen due to various reasons, including

>> **Emergency situations,** in which you must spend the time when you would usually sleep in the waiting room of a hospital, for example

>> **Work schedules,** which may interrupt regular sleeping habits if your shift changes or you have to work an increased number of hours

>> **Homework,** which you have put off and now need to pull an all-nighter to complete

>> **Voluntary choices,** such as binge-watching a TV series or reading a thrilling novel until the wee hours of the morning

The effects of acute sleep deprivation are immediate and profound. Without sleep, your brain struggles to function correctly. Studies that use advanced imaging techniques — for example, functional magnetic resonance imaging (fMRI) and positron emission tomography (PET) — have shown that even a single night of sleep deprivation can significantly alter the areas in your brain responsible for

>> **Mood regulation:** In this case, sleep deprivation can hinder the ability to control emotions and respond appropriately to situations. The limbic system (made up of several structures beneath the cerebral cortex) takes part in mood regulation, along with the hypothalamus, thalamus, amygdala, and basal ganglia.

>> **Stress response:** Lack of adequate sleep can interfere with the important fight-or-flight response to stress by diminishing your ability to quickly and correctly respond to minor and major daily stressors. It involves multiple brain areas, including the amygdala, hippocampus, and prefrontal cortex areas of the brain.

>> **Attention:** Because of excess daytime sleepiness, you can have significant difficulty staying focused on tasks or keeping vigilant in your daily routines. The main area of the brain responsible for keeping you focused is the prefrontal cortex.

>> **Memory:** Your ability to recall information, particularly in the short-term, may be disrupted due to lack of sleep. Multiple areas of the brain work together to process and store various types of memories. For example, the hippocampus is key for forming new memories, and the prefrontal cortex manages short-term working memory.

Figure 3-2 shows these areas of the brain that are affected by sleep deprivation, and the section "Effects on the brain, mind, and mental health" later in the chapter goes into more detail about how the lack of sleep affects your mood, emotions, focus, and memories.

REMEMBER

Sleep deprivation can have physiological as well as behavioral consequences — from impacts to your physical health to effects on your daily performance and relationships. For example, you might find yourself feeling irritable, overly emotional, or struggling to concentrate on simple tasks.

Moreover, sleep-deprived individuals often experience an increased propensity for daytime sleepiness. This is not just a feeling of being tired; it's a measurable reduction in your ability to stay awake and alert. Tools such as the Multiple Sleep Latency Test (MSLT) and the Maintenance of Wakefulness Test (MWT) objectively measure how quickly a person falls asleep or is able to maintain wakefulness during the day, respectively (turn to Chapter 7 to read more about these objective tests that sleep specialists use to assess sleepiness). Results from these tests consistently show that those who are sleep deprived fall asleep much faster and have a rebound of NREM and REM sleep during these tests.

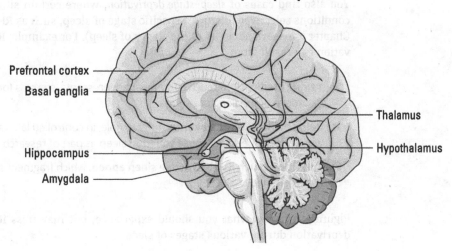

Brain Areas Affected by Sleep Deprivation

Prefrontal cortex

Basal ganglia

Thalamus

Hypothalamus

Hippocampus

Amygdala

FIGURE 3-2:
Areas of the brain that can be affected by sleep deprivation.

WARNING

Acute sleep deprivation can also impair higher-order executive functions, such as decision-making and problem-solving. Tasks that require continuous attention, such as driving, become hazardous. Your reaction times slow down, memory recall becomes fuzzy, and your ability to process complex information diminishes. These impairments can lead to poor judgment and increased risk of accidents, which makes acute sleep deprivation a serious concern.

Partial and sleep-stage deprivation

Partial sleep deprivation occurs when you reduce your total sleep time, getting less sleep than usual but not entirely eliminating it. This situation can be due to

>> **Lifestyle choices:** For example, you aren't making sleep a priority, and wake up early every day to work out or stay up late every night because you enjoy how quiet it is.

>> **Work commitments:** You may find, for example, that — due to a deadline at work — you are curtailing your sleep for a few nights to meet it.

>> **Poor sleep habits:** You take a long nap a few times a week, despite these naps making it difficult for you to sleep well at night.

REMEMBER

Partial sleep deprivation can manifest as not getting the usual amount of sleep that you need to be refreshed in the morning. While this partial deprivation might not seem as severe as complete sleep deprivation, its effects can accumulate over time and lead to significant impairments.

You also find cases of *sleep-stage deprivation*, where certain situations or health conditions selectively disrupt a specific stage of sleep, such as REM sleep (turn to Chapter 2 to learn about all of the stages of sleep). For example, REM sleep deprivation can result from

>> **Taking medications,** such as some antidepressants, steroids for immune disorders, or inhalers for asthma

>> **Being deliberately awakened,** for example, in controlled laboratory settings where sleep specialists rouse you from sleep as part of research sleep studies

>> **Conditions such as obstructive sleep apnea,** which fragment sleep especially in REM sleep

Figure 3-3 shows what you should experience, but may miss if you have sleep deprivation during various stages of sleep.

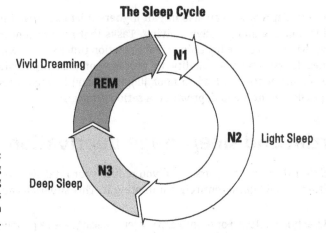

The Sleep Cycle

FIGURE 3-3: Missing sleep during different stages impacts you in different ways.

The consequences of partial and sleep-stage deprivation are subtle yet pervasive. In terms of physical health, partial sleep deprivation can lead to a range of issues, from metabolic disruptions to immune system impairments. And you may notice

>> **Increased sleepiness during the day** in situations where ordinarily you would be able to stay awake, such as working on the computer or during a meeting.

>> **Mood disturbances such as irritability** that affect how you are able to respond to normal day-to-day challenges or during interactions with coworkers or family members.

>> **Riskier decision-making** that is due to impaired judgment and loss of impulse control

>> **Decline in cognitive functions,** particularly *memory consolidation* (the process by which short-term memories become long-term memories), which primarily occurs during deep sleep and REM sleep, leading to difficulties in learning and retaining new information

For more information about memory consolidation, see the section "Recognizing the Physiological Consequences of Inadequate Sleep" later in this chapter.

WARNING

Even a slight reduction in sleep can have a significant impact on your overall health. Researchers have linked chronic partial sleep deprivation to an increased risk of obesity, diabetes, and cardiovascular diseases.

Chronic sleep loss and fragmentation

Chronic sleep loss, also known as *sleep restriction*, occurs when you consistently get less sleep than your body needs over an extended period. In the field of sleep medicine, this situation is also referred to as *chronic volitional sleep restriction* or *insufficient sleep syndrome*. Unlike *acute sleep deprivation*, which is a short-term lack of sleep, chronic sleep loss can last weeks, months, or even years. This condition is often the result of lifestyle factors, work schedules, or medical conditions that prevent sufficient sleep.

Sleep fragmentation is a form of chronic sleep loss where frequent awakenings interrupt your sleep and cause your sleep quality to decrease. Sleep fragmentation can be due to sleep disorders such as sleep apnea or periodic limb movement disorder, or it can result from environmental factors such as noise or an uncomfortable sleeping arrangement. These constant sleep disruptions prevent your body from reaching and maintaining deeper stages of sleep, which are crucial for physical and mental restoration.

The effects of chronic sleep loss are cumulative and can be severe (I cover these effects in more detail in the section "Recognizing the Physiological Consequences of Inadequate Sleep" later in the chapter). Over time, chronic sleep loss can lead to

>> **Significant impairments in cognitive functions,** including attention, memory, and executive functioning

>> **Increased risk of developing mood disorders** such as depression and anxiety

>> **High stress levels,** which make it harder for you to cope with typical daily challenges

Chronic sleep loss and fragmentation not only affect your day-to-day functioning, but also pose long-term health risks. From a physiological perspective, chronic sleep loss can lead to

» **Metabolic disturbances,** such as insulin resistance, an increased risk of type 2 diabetes, and increased weight gain

» **A weakened immune system,** which makes you more susceptible to infections

» **Compromised cardiovascular health,** with increased risks of hypertension, heart disease, and stroke

TIP

Look for practical solutions to manage your sleep and avoid deprivation; get the rest you need to live a healthy, balanced life. See the section "Managing Your Sleep to Avoid Deprivation and Loss" later in the chapter. And begin by prioritizing sleep and addressing any factors that contribute to chronic sleep deprivation to maintain your overall well-being.

Finding Out How and Why Sleep Loss Occurs

Many factors can influence sleep loss, from environmental conditions to underlying health issues. In this section, I help you explore how various factors such as lighting, temperature, and noise in your sleep environment can disrupt sleep, as well as how medical conditions and medications might contribute to sleep problems. Understanding the root causes of sleep loss is the first step in addressing and managing these issues effectively.

Environmental factors affecting sleep

Environmental factors can play a significant role in your sleep quality and duration. Among these, lighting is particularly influential. Light exposure, especially blue light from screens, can interfere with your *circadian rhythm* — the internal clock that regulates sleep-wake cycles (see Chapter 7 for more information). The circadian system is highly sensitive to light, and exposing yourself to light at the wrong times can cause your body to delay producing melatonin, the hormone that promotes sleepiness.

Managing light

Psychiatrists and psychologists may prescribe light therapy for patients with seasonal affective disorder (SAD), while sleep specialists often prescribe light therapy to treat conditions of certain circadian rhythm disorders (see Chapter 7) in their patients, helping them to realign their sleep patterns with their preferred schedule.

WARNING

Always follow your sleep specialist's guidance about how and when to use light therapy because improper timing can further disrupt your sleep. Also, getting the proper settings to use for light wavelength, intensity, timing, and distance from the light box is important. The timing and settings are all specific to you as an individual, so make sure to follow all instructions for optimal treatment.

Maintaining the right temperature

Temperature also affects your sleep. Your body's core temperature naturally drops during sleep, reaching its lowest point in the early morning. This temperature drop is crucial in helping you fall and stay asleep. Fluctuations in environmental temperature can disrupt this process.

TIP

Ideally, your sleeping environment should be cool, but not cold, to promote restful sleep. Studies suggest that warming up, perhaps by taking a warm bath before bed, can help you fall asleep better by accelerating your body's heat loss process. Because of the warm bath, the blood vessels close to the skin dilate and facilitate the natural drop in your core body temperature.

Nixing the noise

Noise is another critical factor. Although some people find white noise or soft music soothing while sleeping, unwanted noises can be disruptive. Chronic exposure to noise, such as traffic, aircraft, or industrial sounds, can lead to sleep disturbances and even long-term health issues — cardiovascular disease, for example.

The World Health Organization estimates that people lose millions of healthy life years annually due to noise-related sleep disturbances. It's not just the volume of noise but also the unpredictability that can be jarring. Consistent, predictable sounds are less likely to wake you up than sudden, intermittent noises.

Neurologic, psychiatric, and other disorders affecting sleep

In Chapters 7 and 8, I go into great detail about the causes, effects, diagnoses, and treatment of sleep disorders — head to those chapters if you'd like to read about that in depth. In this section, I cover several medical conditions that can significantly impact your sleep quality and duration.

Insomnia and other sleep disorders

Fragmentation of sleep resulting from sleep disorders not only reduces your overall sleep quality but also results in daytime sleepiness and increases the risk of severe health issues, including hypertension, cardiovascular disease, and diabetes. Here are some of the sleep disorders that can contribute to sleep deprivation and loss:

>> *Insomnia* is one of the most common sleep disorders, in which you have difficulty falling asleep or staying asleep, or you wake up too soon. Insomnia results in sleep loss that, in turn, can cause you to experience significant daytime impairment, including mood disturbances and cognitive deficits.

Sleep specialists often recognize a link between insomnia and psychiatric conditions such as depression and anxiety. This link creates a cycle where each condition exacerbates the other.

>> *Obstructive sleep apnea* (OSA) is another prevalent condition, which occurs when a person's airway becomes partially or completely blocked during sleep. This situation leads to brief but frequent awakenings as your body struggles to breathe. The OSA condition affects approximately 24 percent of men and 9 percent of women between the ages of 30 and 60 years. These rates are higher for individuals who are obese.

>> *Shift work sleep disorder* affects individuals who work nontraditional hours, such as night shifts or rotating shifts. The disorder results from the misalignment between a person's internal clock and their work schedule.

This noted misalignment can lead to chronic sleep deprivation and a host of related problems, including increased risk of motor vehicle and work-related accidents, mood disturbances, and long-term health consequences such as gastrointestinal issues and cardiovascular disease.

>> *Restless legs syndrome* (RLS) is another condition that can result in sleep loss. Individuals with RLS experience uncomfortable sensations in their legs, often described as tingling, crawling, or simply an irresistible urge to move their legs. These sensations can only be relieved by voluntarily moving the legs. If you experience RLS and the constant need to move, you may find falling and staying asleep challenging, and you may suffer from chronic sleep deprivation and its associated consequences.

About 80 percent of those who have RLS also have periodic limb movements during sleep (PLMS), which are typically leg movements that rhythmically occur during sleep and result in further sleep loss due to fragmentation of sleep.

Other physical disorders

Other disorders, such as asthma, chronic obstructive pulmonary disease (COPD), and gastroesophageal reflux disease (GERD), can also impact sleep. These conditions often involve symptoms that worsen at night, such as coughing, wheezing, or acid reflux, leading to frequent awakenings and reduced sleep quality.

Similarly, metabolic disorders — such as diabetes and thyroid disease — can interfere with sleep patterns, either because of their direct symptoms or via the medications used for their treatment.

Medications and other substances that affect sleep

Various medications can impact your sleep, either as a primary effect or as a side effect:

>> **Steroids,** which doctors often prescribe for inflammatory conditions, can disrupt your sleep by causing you agitation and restlessness. Patients with conditions such as asthma who use corticosteroids frequently report insomnia.

>> **Caffeine and theophylline,** which you can commonly find in coffee, tea, and certain medications, are stimulants that can significantly affect your sleep. Although these effects are no secret, I would be remiss not to mention them. These stimulants work by blocking adenosine receptors, which then promotes wakefulness.

REMEMBER

Millions of people regularly consume coffee, soda, energy drinks, and other products to battle daytime drowsiness, but be aware that caffeine's effects can linger for hours and lead to difficulty falling asleep. Theophylline — used in treating respiratory conditions such as asthma — has similar stimulating effects.

>> **Decongestants** can sometimes keep you awake at night, which is such a catch-22. When you have a cold and can't sleep because you can't breathe, you take a decongestant to relieve your nasal blockage, but then you can't sleep because of the stimulants in some of these medications!

>> **Medications containing pseudoephedrine** can increase your heart rate and cause feelings of anxiety or restlessness, which then makes falling asleep harder.

>> **Cardiovascular medications** can affect your sleep in various ways. Beta-blockers, which you may use to manage hypertension and other heart conditions, can reduce your body's melatonin production, leading to insomnia.

TIP

Not all beta-blockers reduce melatonin production. Carvedilol and nebivolol are options that don't have this negative effect.

» **Stimulants prescribed for conditions such as attention-deficit hyperactivity disorder (ADHD) or narcolepsy** can improve your wakefulness during the day, but may make it hard for you to sleep if you take them too late in the day. If you use these medications — for example, amphetamines or methylphenidate — adhere to the instructions in your prescription, including the timing of your doses, to balance daytime alertness with nighttime sleep quality.

Substance abuse can also play a significant role in sleep disturbances:

» **Alcohol** might seem to be a great sleeping tool, but it's a trick. It can initially sedate you deeply and swiftly — which seems helpful for falling asleep — but it can disrupt your *sleep architecture* (the structure of sleep cycles and stages that you experience throughout the night) and result in lighter, fragmented sleep. As your body metabolizes alcohol, you wake frequently and get less REM sleep.

» **Nicotine** in cigarettes has a similar dual effect. While it can be relaxing initially, it's a stimulant that can cause insomnia, especially in habitual smokers who experience withdrawal symptoms during the night.

Recognizing the Physiological Consequences of Inadequate Sleep

Sleep is not just a luxury — it's a vital component of good health. Inadequate sleep can wreak havoc on various bodily systems, leading to a range of physiological consequences. This section focuses on the impact of sleep deprivation on your brain, metabolism, immune function, and cardiovascular health. From cognitive impairments and mood disorders to metabolic and immune dysfunctions, the effects of sleep loss are far-reaching and can have significant effects on your overall health.

Effects on the brain, mind, and mental health

Inadequate sleep significantly impacts your brain's ability to function optimally and guide you in various aspects of your life. Lack of sleep is an impairment that results in slower reaction times and decreased accuracy. You may find that focusing on essential tasks or picking out critical information in a hectic environment is more difficult. And although you may not have trouble forming new memories when you're sleep deprived, you might be less effective at the process of stabilizing and retaining these memories over time.

Researchers have also linked chronic sleep deprivation to heightened stress responses, because your body's ability to manage stress diminishes without adequate rest. Also, your ability to sustain and manage your activities in social and work situations can suffer when you're sleep deprived.

About paying attention

One of the most immediate adverse effects involves *sustained attention*, which is the ability to maintain focus and concentration for an extended period of time. This ability is crucial for completing tasks that require a prolonged focus. When you're sleep deprived, maintaining focus can become challenging and lead to frequent lapses and decreased overall performance. This decline in sustained attention can manifest as difficulty staying on task during meetings, while reading, or when attempting other activities that require continuous mental effort.

Lack of sleep also compromises your *selective attention*, the ability to concentrate on specific stimuli while filtering out distractions. For instance, if you're trying to work in a noisy office when you're sleep deprived, you might find it hard to ignore background chatter and concentrate on work, leading you to make errors and reduce your work efficiency.

Trouble processing memories

In addition to attention-related issues, your memory consolidation — particularly for *declarative memories* (facts, experiences, and events) — suffers if you're not getting enough sleep. This impairment can lead to difficulties in learning new information or recalling previously learned material, which is critical for academic and professional performance. Refer to the section "Acute sleep deprivation" earlier in the chapter and to Figure 3-2 to find out the specific areas in the brain that are responsible for attention and memory processes.

Aggravation to mental health issues

On the mental health front, if you have existing mood disorders such as depression and anxiety, sleep deprivation can exacerbate them. The relationship between sleep and mood is bidirectional, meaning poor sleep can worsen symptoms of these conditions, while these conditions can, in turn, disrupt sleep, as depicted in Figure 3-4.

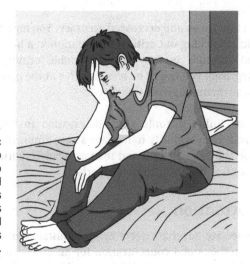

FIGURE 3-4:
The relationship
between sleep
deprivation and
mood disorders
(such as
depression and
anxiety) is
bidirectional .

WARNING

Sleep loss lowers your threshold for experiencing negative emotions, making you more prone to irritability and emotional instability when you're sleep deprived.

Inhibiting social relationships

Sleep deprivation doesn't just affect your emotional and mental health; it also has significant *psychosocial* impacts. That is, the way you interact with others and per-ceive social situations can be profoundly influenced by how well rested you are. When you don't get enough sleep, you're more likely to experience:

>> **Emotional reactivity:** Studies have shown that sleep-deprived individuals are more likely to overreact to minor annoyances and experience mood swings. This increased emotional volatility can strain personal and professional relationships, making it challenging to communicate effectively and resolve conflicts.

>> **Reduced empathy:** Sleep deprivation can dull your ability to empathize with others. Empathy is crucial for understanding and sharing the feelings of others, whether it's in a family setting, workplace, or social environment. When you're tired, you may find it harder to interpret social cues and respond compassionately, leading to misunderstandings and decreased social support.

>> **Impaired social judgment:** Decision-making isn't just about logic and facts; it also involves understanding social dynamics and the potential consequences of your actions. Sleep deprivation can impair your social judgment, making it difficult to assess situations accurately. You may find yourself making poor decisions that result in unfortunate actions — such as an off-base response triggered by misjudging the tone of an email or reacting inappropriately to a colleague's comment. These situations can lead to unnecessary conflicts.

- **Loneliness and social isolation:** The effects of sleep deprivation can also contribute to feelings of loneliness and social isolation. When you're constantly tired, you're less likely to engage in social activities and more likely to withdraw from social interactions. This withdrawal can create a cycle where reduced social engagement leads to further feelings of loneliness, which can, in turn, exacerbate sleep problems.

- **Impact on family and intimate relationships:** Sleep deprivation can strain intimate relationships. Partners may experience irritability and reduced patience with each other, leading to increased arguments and decreased relationship satisfaction. Lack of sleep can also affect libido and intimacy, which can further strain relationships.

- **Workplace dynamics:** In a professional setting, sleep-deprived employees may struggle with teamwork and collaboration. Mood changes can lead to conflicts with colleagues, and impaired decision-making can affect team performance. Additionally, sleep-deprived leaders may be less effective in managing their teams, which can lead to a less productive and more stressful work environment.

TIP

If sleep deprivation is affecting your relationships or social life, consider seeking support from a sleep specialist with experience in psychiatry or psychology. This expertise can be particularly effective for addressing both sleep issues and the psychosocial challenges associated with them.

Mitigating adverse effects of sleep deprivation

To mitigate cognitive, mental, emotional, and psychosocial impacts of sleep deprivation, it's crucial to prioritize good sleep hygiene (or habits). Simple practices such as maintaining a regular sleep schedule, creating a relaxing bedtime routine, and minimizing screen time before bed can make a significant difference. (Turn to Chapter 15 for more details and tips on how to build and maintain great sleep practices!) Additionally, monitoring your emotional state and taking proactive steps to manage stress — such as practicing mindfulness or engaging in regular physical activity — can help improve both sleep quality and social interactions.

REMEMBER

To maintain your mental health, care for your sleep by

- **Practicing mindfulness and relaxation techniques:** Try meditation, deep breathing exercises, and progressive muscle relaxation before bed. These techniques can help manage stress and anxiety if you feel they are impacting your sleep, by promoting better sleep and mental well-being. High achievers in particular may benefit from mindfulness to maintain focus and calm during big work events, competitions, and other major milestones.

>> **Exploring cognitive behavioral therapy for insomnia (CBT-I):** CBT-I is a proven method to address chronic insomnia and improve sleep quality. This therapy focuses on many different treatments, including changing negative thought patterns and behaviors that contribute to sleep loss, offering a structured approach to improving sleep. (For more on how CBT-I works, turn to Chapter 7.)

Effects on metabolic, endocrine, and immune systems

Sleep plays a crucial role in regulating your metabolic processes. For example, when you don't get enough sleep, the hormones that control your hunger and appetite become dysregulated. Your endocrine system, which includes glands that produce hormones, also suffers from lack of sleep. And adequate sleep is essential for maintaining a healthy immune system and proper functioning of the body's basic systems that manage your breathing, blood flow, and digestion.

Fueling your body for sleep

WARNING

Sleep deprivation increases levels of *ghrelin*, the hormone that stimulates hunger, while it decreases levels of *leptin*, the hormone that signals satiety. This imbalance causes your appetite to increase, particularly for high-calorie, carbohydrate-rich foods, which could possibly contribute to weight gain and obesity, as depicted in Figure 3-5.

Imbalanced Hunger Hormones

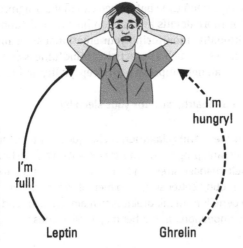

I'm hungry!

I'm full!

Leptin

Ghrelin

FIGURE 3-5:
Sleep deprivation leads to changes in the hormones ghrelin and leptin, which can lead you to feel hungrier than you actually are.

On the other side of the coin, managing your food intake wisely can actually help you sleep:

>> **Avoid eating large meals too close to bedtime** by trying to eat nothing during the two to three hours before bedtime.

>> **Avoid caffeine, alcohol, and high-sugar snacks** at dinner or in the evening.

>> **Try specific foods when you do eat dinner** or have something in the evening. You may consider reaching for foods high in tryptophan (for example, turkey and nuts) or foods rich in magnesium (such as leafy greens and bananas). However, the evidence that these foods help in promoting sleep is mixed.

>> **Eat smaller, balanced meals throughout the day** to stabilize your blood sugar levels, which can help you prevent sleep disruptions caused by hunger or indigestion.

Keeping your hormones in order

The fact is that your body's production of cortisol, a hormone associated with stress, follows a daily rhythm that sleep deprivation disrupts. Elevated cortisol levels can lead to a range of issues, including increased stress, anxiety, and difficulties in regulating blood sugar levels.

WARNING

Inadequate sleep is particularly concerning if you have or are at risk of developing type 2 diabetes, because sleep deprivation reduces insulin sensitivity, making it harder for you to manage blood glucose levels, which is important to thwart diabetes.

Supporting your immune system

Your immune system also suffers when you get inadequate sleep. Sleep is essential for the production of *cytokines*, which are proteins that help fight infections and inflammation. When you're sleep-deprived, your body produces fewer cytokines, which weakens your immune response. This reduction makes you more susceptible to infections such as the common cold and can prolong recovery times.

REMEMBER

Researchers have also linked chronic sleep deprivation to chronic inflammation, which is a risk factor for a variety of diseases, including cardiovascular disease, cancer, and neurodegenerative disorders.

Effects on the cardiovascular and other systems

Sleep is a fundamental pillar of health that influences almost every system in your body. When you don't get enough sleep, the consequences ripple through your cardiovascular, respiratory, gastrointestinal, musculoskeletal, and reproductive systems, leading to a variety of serious health issues. From increasing your risk of heart disease to exacerbating conditions such as asthma, the effects of sleep deprivation can be profound and far-reaching.

Cardiovascular system

Not getting enough sleep keeps your body in a constant state of alertness, which puts extra pressure on your heart and blood vessels. This prolonged stress can damage your cardiovascular system, increasing the likelihood of serious health problems. Researchers have linked inadequate sleep to a range of cardiovascular risks, including

>> **Hypertension, or high blood pressure:** A condition in which the pressure in your blood vessels is consistently higher than age-adjusted normal ranges. This condition contributes to an increased risk of diseases of the heart, brain, and kidneys.

>> **Heart disease:** This category covers various conditions that affect the heart muscle and valves, and/or the associated arteries. Examples include coronary artery disease, congestive heart failure, and arrhythmias.

>> **Stroke:** A condition that results in damage to brain tissue when blood flow to the brain is abruptly reduced or sudden bleeding happens in the brain.

These cardiovascular risks can arise partially because sleep deprivation activates the sympathetic nervous system, which is responsible for your body's *fight-or-flight response* (an instinctive physiological response to a threat). This system prepares your body to deal with stress or danger by increasing your heart rate and blood pressure.

WARNING

When you're sleep deprived, this stress response becomes more active even when you're at rest. This means your heart has to work harder than usual and increases your blood pressure, even if you're not doing anything physically demanding. Over time, this constant strain can cause your blood vessels to stiffen and narrow.

Another pathway in the cardiovascular systems that may be affected is the *endothelial cells*, which line the blood vessels. Sleep loss and mental stress can cause dysfunction of these cells and lead to the buildup of plaque — a mix of fat, cholesterol, and other substances — inside the arteries. The resulting condition is called *atherosclerosis,* and is depicted in Figure 3-6.

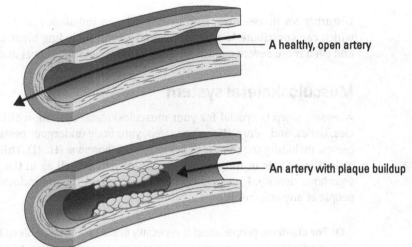

A healthy, open artery

An artery with plaque buildup

FIGURE 3-6:
The buildup of
plaque in once
healthy
blood vessels.

This plaque buildup can result in blood clots that either remain in the blood vessels and block them (thrombi) or break off and travel to another body location such as the brain or heart (emboli). This process increases your risk of heart attacks and strokes because your heart and brain may not get enough oxygen-rich blood as a result of these thrombi or emboli.

Respiratory system

Sleep deprivation also impacts respiratory function, especially if you have preexisting conditions such as asthma or chronic obstructive pulmonary disease (COPD). Sleep loss can exacerbate related symptoms, such as shortness of breath and wheezing, and lead to more frequent nighttime awakenings and poorer overall sleep quality. This disruption can create a vicious cycle, where inadequate sleep worsens respiratory symptoms, which in turn further impairs sleep.

Gastrointestinal system

Sleep deprivation can have a notable impact on the gastrointestinal system. One of the lesser-known consequences is its potential to exacerbate conditions such as *gastroesophageal reflux disease* (GERD). Lack of sleep can increase acid production in your stomach, leading to more frequent and severe episodes of acid reflux. This condition can cause discomfort and further disrupt sleep, creating a vicious cycle.

Moreover, researchers have linked sleep deprivation to altered *gut microbiota* — the community of microorganisms living in the digestive tract. A healthy gut microbiome is essential for digestion, nutrient absorption, and immune function.

Disturbances in sleep can lead to *dysbiosis*, an imbalance in the gut microbiota, which can contribute to gastrointestinal issues, including bloating, constipation, and even more severe conditions such as inflammatory bowel disease (IBD).

Musculoskeletal system

Adequate sleep is crucial for your musculoskeletal system, which includes muscles, bones, and joints. When you sleep, your body undergoes essential repair processes, including the release of *human growth hormone* (HGH). This hormone plays a significant role in muscle repair and growth, as well as in the maintenance of your bone density. Lack of proper sleep can affect the musculoskeletal system of people at any stage of life:

>> **For children,** proper sleep is especially important because sleep loss can result in less HGH secretion, which in turn can result in delayed growth.

>> **For any active person,** when you don't get enough sleep, you are slower to recover from injuries, experience increased muscle soreness, and are at a higher risk of musculoskeletal injuries. This means sleep is extremely important for athletes in particular!

>> **For people as they age,** chronic sleep deprivation can contribute to osteoporosis by affecting the balance of *bone remodeling,* the process where old bone tissue is replaced with new tissue. A lack of sleep can disrupt the balance of hormones involved in this process — such as cortisol and *parathyroid hormone* — potentially leading to decreased bone density over time.

Reproductive system

Sleep deprivation can also wreak havoc on your reproductive system.

>> **For men,** sleep deprivation can reduce testosterone levels, which can affect libido, muscle mass, and overall energy levels. You primarily produce testosterone during sleep, and insufficient rest can lead to lower production levels, impacting reproductive health and well-being.

>> **For women,** irregular sleep patterns can disrupt the menstrual cycle and affect fertility. If you're not getting enough sleep, you may experience hormonal imbalances, including fluctuations in estrogen and progesterone levels. These imbalances can not only affect menstrual regularity but can also exacerbate symptoms of premenstrual syndrome (PMS) and other hormonal conditions.

Detecting Behavioral Consequences of Inadequate Sleep

Lack of sleep doesn't affect only your physical health; it can significantly alter your behavior and daily performance. From the dangers of drowsy driving to the impact on job performance and athletic abilities, the behavioral consequences of sleep deprivation are far-reaching.

Effects on driving

WARNING

Driving while sleep-deprived can be as dangerous as driving under the influence of alcohol. Drowsy driving impairs your ability to react quickly to situations you encounter on the road, such as a car stopping suddenly or a pedestrian crossing in front of you.

Sleep deprivation has these effects:

>> It slows down your reaction times, which are critical to defensive driving.

>> It reduces your ability to remain alert to ever-changing driving conditions.

>> It decreases your ability to focus on the task at hand — in this case, driving safely.

REMEMBER

Studies show that being awake for 18 hours straight impairs your driving ability to the same extent as having a blood alcohol concentration (BAC) of 0.05 percent, and staying awake for 24 hours equates to a BAC of 0.10 percent, which is over the legal limit for driving in many places.

Watching out for microsleeps

One of the most dangerous aspects of drowsy driving is the occurrence of microsleeps, which can happen without warning, even when your eyes are open. The risk of microsleeps increases with the severity of sleep deprivation and is particularly common during monotonous activities such as long-distance driving on highways.

WARNING

During a microsleep, you're essentially driving blind, which can lead to catastrophic personal and public health consequences, especially if you're traveling at high speed.

Having increased risk from a sleep disorder

Sleep disorders such as OSA or hypersomnia further exacerbate the risks associated with drowsy driving. If you have OSA or hypersomnia, you're more prone to day-time sleepiness, which increases your likelihood of experiencing microsleeps while driving. As a result, you have a higher risk of being involved in traffic accidents.

TIP

If you have OSA, hypersomnia, or any sleep disorder, seek treatment at a sleep center and be cautious about driving (for example, have someone else drive, especially for long distances) when you haven't had adequate rest.

Effects on job performance

As a surprise to probably no one, sleep-deprived individuals often aren't as pro-ductive or accurate at work as their well-rested coworkers due to the decline in cognitive functions such as attention, memory, and decision-making. Most peo-ple have probably gone to work tired at some point — for whatever reason — and you may be familiar with some effects that can happen when you haven't gotten enough sleep:

>> **Impaired cognitive function can occur.** You can struggle to focus on tasks, might miss critical details, and make poor decisions. Sometimes you can get through your workday in this state, but if you're in a profession that requires quick decisions and complex tasks (for example, air traffic controller, surgeon, or firefighter), mistakes can have severe consequences — even up to injury or death.

>> **Physical performance can also suffer.** For workers in physically demanding jobs, such as construction or emergency services, inadequate sleep can lead to slower reaction times, decreased coordination, and increased risk of injuries.

>> **Communication and teamwork can become difficult.** Sleep deprivation can also impair the ability to communicate effectively and work as part of a team, which is crucial in many job settings.

REMEMBER

Specific populations, such as military personnel and medical residents, are often at a higher risk of sleep deprivation due to the demanding nature of their work schedules. These groups have been the subject of several research studies, and they may experience chronic sleep deprivation, leading to burnout, decreased job satisfaction, and higher rates of mental health issues such as depression and anxiety.

If you're a shift worker with a rotating schedule, maintaining a consistent sleep routine can be challenging. However, these strategies can help you ease the tran-sition and improve your sleep quality:

>> **Gradual adjustments:** Before a shift change, gradually adjust your sleep schedule by shifting your bedtime and wake time by an hour or two each day. This slow adjustment helps your body acclimate to the new schedule more smoothly.

>> **Consistent sleep schedule:** On your days off, try to maintain a consistent sleep schedule that closely aligns with your workdays. This consistency helps regulate your body's internal clock and reduces the strain of constantly shifting your sleep patterns.

>> **Light exposure management:** Use light exposure strategically to help adjust your circadian rhythm (Chapters 4 and 7 have more information on circadian rhythm). Seek bright light exposure during your waking hours, whether through natural sunlight or artificial light therapy. Conversely, wear sunglasses during your commute home if it's daylight to reduce light exposure and signal to your body that it's time to wind down. Try to avoid any bright light in your home since it can delay your onset of sleep.

>> **Open communication:** Inform family and friends about your work and sleep schedule, and ask for their understanding and support in minimizing disturbances during your designated sleep times. Setting boundaries and communicating your needs can help create a more supportive environment for restful sleep.

>> **Napping strategies:** If you find it difficult to get a full sleep session in one go, consider strategic napping. A short nap (20 minutes, for example) before your shift can help boost alertness and performance. However, avoid napping too close to your main sleep period to prevent disrupting your sleep cycle.

TIP

If you're a manager, addressing sleep deprivation in the workplace through policies like appropriate shift scheduling and sleep education can help mitigate these risks and improve overall job performance and safety for your employees.

Effects on athletic performance

Athletes, both professional and recreational, can experience significant declines in performance due to inadequate sleep. Without sufficient rest, athletes may find it challenging to maintain peak physical condition because sleep deprivation can lead to decreased strength, slower reaction times, and reduced endurance.

Sleep deprivation can affect these aspects of athletic performance:

>> **Your body's circadian rhythm,** which regulates the timing of various physiological processes, including those related to exercise and sleep. If you're an athlete and your circadian rhythm gets disrupted, perhaps by late-night

training sessions or travel across time zones, your performance may suffer. For instance, your peak performance time may shift, making it harder to achieve optimal results during games and competitions when they happen at atypical times.

>> **Your motor skills and coordination** can suffer, which can lead to a higher risk of injuries. Fine motor skills, such as those you need in sports such as gymnastics or tennis, can become less precise, while gross motor skills, like those you use in running or jumping, can also deteriorate.

>> **Mental aspects of performance,** such as focus, motivation, and emotional regulation, are equally important. Sleep-deprived athletes may struggle to stay motivated, manage stress, and maintain a positive mindset, all of which are crucial for success in sports.

If you're an athlete who wants to get enough sleep, you should

>> **Establish a consistent sleep routine:** Maintaining a regular sleep schedule, even on weekends, helps regulate the body's internal clock and can improve both the quality and duration of sleep. You should aim for seven to nine hours of sleep per night, depending on your individual needs and training intensity.

>> **Create a sleep-friendly environment:** Ensuring a quiet, dark, and cool sleeping environment can enhance sleep quality. Aside from making sure your pillows and mattress are to your liking, consider using blackout curtains, earplugs, or white noise machines to block out disturbances.

>> **Manage pre-competition anxiety:** Anxiety and excitement before competitions can interfere with sleep. Try relaxation techniques such as deep breathing, meditation, or progressive muscle relaxation to calm your mind before bed. Avoiding stimulating activities, including intense exercise or screen use, one to two hours before sleep can also help.

>> **Optimize nutrition and hydration:** Consume a balanced diet with adequate protein and carbohydrates to support your body's recovery and energy levels while you sleep. Avoid caffeine and heavy meals close to bedtime because these can disrupt your sleep.

>> **Plan for travel and time zone changes:** When you travel across time zones, adjust your sleep schedule in advance to help minimize jet lag. If you can, gradually shift sleep and wake times in advance to align with your destination's time zone to help ease your transition. Alternatively, arrive early at your destination by a few days to adjust to the new time zone. Also, light exposure management — such as seeking sunlight in the morning and avoiding bright light in the evening — can also aid in adjusting your circadian rhythm.

Effects on specific groups of people

Other groups of individuals that are more vulnerable to the effects of sleep deprivation due to specific circumstances include

>> **Parents of young children:** They often experience interrupted sleep, which can lead to chronic sleep deprivation. This population not only faces the immediate challenges of being alert and responsive to a child's needs, but also deals with the long-term consequences of insufficient rest — such as decreased immune function and heightened stress levels.

>> **Older adults:** As people age and experience the normal effects of age on sleep quality and quantity (and the increased prevalence of medical and sleep disorders that can result in sleep loss), they often experience a decrease in deep sleep and an increase in nighttime awakenings. This sleep fragmentation can exacerbate other issues associated with aging, such as cognitive decline and increased risk of falls.

>> **College students:** The culture of late-night studying and early morning classes can lead to a chronic state of sleep deficit, impairing memory consolidation and learning. This population may resort to stimulants like caffeine or energy drinks to stay awake, which can further disrupt their sleep patterns.

THE ECONOMIC IMPACT OF SLEEP DEPRIVATION

The economic impact of sleep deprivation extends beyond personal health and well-being. It has far-reaching consequences for productivity, healthcare costs, and workplace safety. In the United States alone, sleep deprivation costs the economy up to approximately $411 billion annually due to these factors:

- Lost productivity from *absenteeism* (absence from work for lengths beyond what is considered a typically acceptable) and *presenteeism* (present but not fully functioning in the workplace).

- Decline in productivity that leads to missed deadlines, poor decision-making, and a general decrease in work quality. Employees who don't get enough sleep are more likely to experience decreased concentration, slower reaction times, and an increased likelihood of making errors. Companies may face higher operational costs due to the need for additional staffing, overtime pay, and error correction.

- Increased healthcare expenses and occurrence of accidents.

(continued)

(continued)

Chronic sleep deprivation is linked to various health conditions, including cardiovascular diseases, diabetes, and mental health disorders. These conditions require medical intervention, increasing the demand for healthcare services and raising insurance premiums. Moreover, sleep-deprived individuals are more likely to require frequent medical consultations and medications, which further strains the healthcare system.

Sleep deprivation contributes to a significant number of workplace accidents, especially in industries that require high levels of alertness, such as transportation, construction, and healthcare. The National Highway Traffic Safety Administration (NHTSA) estimates that drowsy driving is responsible for approximately 72,000 crashes annually in the U.S. These incidents not only result in loss of life but also lead to legal liabilities, increased insurance costs, and lost productivity due to injuries.

To combat the economic and social impact of sleep deprivation, public health campaigns can play a vital role. These initiatives aim to raise awareness about the importance of sleep, promote good sleep hygiene practices, and encourage employers to create work environments that prioritize employee well-being. For example, flexible work hours, nap rooms, and wellness programs can help mitigate the effects of sleep deprivation and improve overall productivity.

Managing Your Sleep to Avoid Deprivation and Loss

Getting good sleep isn't just about clocking enough hours in bed; it's about ensuring the quality of your sleep. In this section, I give you practical strategies to help manage and optimize your sleep. From the benefits of napping to the use of medications, I offer ideas to help you avoid sleep deprivation and maintain overall well-being. Whether you're dealing with a busy schedule or struggling with sleep issues, these tips can help you get the rest you need.

Are naps and short-term countermeasures for sleep loss useful?

Napping can be a valuable tool to help you manage sleep debt and boost alertness, especially when you can't get a full night's rest. However, how effective your naps are depends on their timing and duration:

>> **Short naps, lasting 10–20 minutes, can help you enhance alertness and improve mood without leaving you groggy.** These quick naps are great for boosting concentration and performance in the short term. To avoid interfering with your nighttime sleep, if you need to take a nap, take it early in the day.

>> **Longer naps, around 90 minutes, may allow you to complete a full sleep cycle, including light sleep, deep sleep, and REM sleep.** While these longer naps can offer more substantial restorative benefits, they may cause you to feel groggy if you wake up during deep sleep (a condition called *sleep inertia*) and are generally not recommended unless you take this nap every day at the same time for the same amount of time.

In addition to naps, other short-term countermeasures can sometimes help you mitigate the effects of sleep deprivation. Caffeine can temporarily boost your alertness and reduce fatigue, but make sure to use it wisely, keeping in mind that too much can lead to tolerance and withdrawal symptoms. Also, caffeine has a half-life of about five to six hours, so avoid consuming it late in the day if you want to sleep well at night.

REMEMBER

If you are driving, blasting the radio or opening the windows have only a very modest and short-term effect on your drowsiness, especially if you are significantly sleep deprived. In this situation, the best approach to tackling your drowsiness is to pull the car over and have someone else drive, or, if you are alone, take a short nap in a safe location.

Light exposure can also help you manage your sleep patterns. Getting plenty of natural sunlight in the morning can help reset your circadian rhythm, making it easier to wake up and stay alert during the day. In the evening, reduce your exposure to blue light from screens to help signal to your body that it's time to wind down.

TIP

While naps and short-term solutions can provide temporary relief from sleep deprivation, prioritize regular, sufficient nighttime sleep to maintain optimal health and well-being.

Over-the-counter and prescribed medications

If you're struggling with sleep issues, over-the-counter (OTC) and prescribed medications might be an option to consider for improving sleep quality. However, always use these medications cautiously and under the guidance of a healthcare professional because they can have side effects and potential for dependency.

OTC options include

>> **Antihistamines:** Some OTC sleep aids contain antihistamines like diphen-hydramine or doxylamine, which can make you drowsy. While these may help you fall asleep, they can also leave you feeling groggy the next day. Use them sparingly and not as a long-term solution, because you may develop *tolerance* to these medications over time (that is, your body metabolizes these medications faster and they gradually lose their effectiveness).

>> **Melatonin:** Sleep aids with melatonin can be helpful if you're adjusting to a new time zone or dealing with delayed sleep phase disorder. Unlike other sleep aids, melatonin doesn't cause dependency, which makes it a safer option for occasional use. Start with a low dose and consult your healthcare provider to find the right amount for you.

Typically, OTC medications do not constitute long-term help because they either become ineffective or have significant side effects. Talking to your doctor about trying prescription medications or seeing a sleep specialist that can address the underlying cause of your sleep problems is your best move. A sleep specialist might recommend prescription medications such as

>> **Benzodiazepines and non-benzodiazepine hypnotics:** Doctors often prescribe medications like zolpidem and eszopiclone for short-term treatment of insomnia. These drugs work by enhancing the effects of gamma-aminobutyric acid (GABA), a neurotransmitter that promotes relaxation and sleep.

Be aware of potential side effects, including next-day drowsiness and cognitive impairments. Long-term use can lead to tolerance, dependence, and withdrawal symptoms. For these reasons and other safety issues, they are generally prescribed by sleep specialists only for acute or transient sleep difficulties.

>> **Antidepressants:** Doctors prescribe some antidepressants, such as trazo-done and mirtazapine, for their sedative properties. These can be especially useful if you experience both depression and insomnia. However, they may also come with side effects such as weight gain and daytime sleepiness.

>> **Prescription stimulants:** For conditions such as narcolepsy, shift work sleep disorder, and sleepiness associated with OSA that is not improved with OSA treatment, certain stimulants — modafinil and armodafinil, for example — can help keep you awake during the day. These medications must be prescribed and monitored over time under careful medical supervision, because they can have side effects such as increased heart rate and anxiety, and may reduce the effectiveness of birth control pills in women.

REMEMBER

In the book's Appendix A, you can find a table that lists FDA-approved medications used to treat various sleep conditions. While medications can help you manage sleep issues, they aren't a substitute for good sleep hygiene practices. Address any underlying causes of sleep problems, such as stress or poor sleep habits, alongside medication use. See Chapter 6 to find out about how much sleep you really need, how to manage it, and how sleep varies by traits such as age and sex.

2

Surveying Sleep Components and Mechanisms

Chapter **4**

Making the Connection: Sleep and Circadian Mechanisms

Your body regulates sleep through complex biological processes, and one of the most important is your *circadian rhythm sleep-wake* mechanism. This internal system keeps your sleep-wake cycle aligned with the 24-hour day, and influences when you feel tired or alert. In this chapter, you can explore how these circadian rhythms guide your sleep patterns and what happens when this internal clock gets out of sync with the external environment (including societal norms) and your preferences. (See Chapter 7 for specifics of circadian rhythm sleep-wake disorders.)

You also find out how sleep impacts various systems in your body, from your nervous and respiratory systems to your cardiovascular health. Understanding these connections reveals why sleep is so crucial for maintaining your overall well-being. And knowing these connections is also important when things go wrong with specific aspects of the anatomy and physiology of your body — and potentially lead to sleep disorders such as obstructive sleep apnea (OSA).

Specifically, I help you dive into the role of neurotransmitters in regulating sleep cycles and focus on how they manage the transitions between NREM (non-rapid eye movement) and REM (rapid eye movement) sleep. Both stages are essential for body restoration, and I explain how imbalances in these stages can lead to sleep disturbances and health risks.

Recognizing How Sleep Interacts with Your Nervous System

Your *nervous system* (consisting of the brain, spinal cord, and nerves that branch off from the spinal cord) plays a central role in managing your sleep cycles, regulating how you transition between sleep and wakefulness. It orchestrates a variety of bodily functions during sleep. Specifically, the *autonomic nervous system* (ANS, part of the nervous system that branches off from the brain and spinal cord) plays a crucial role by regulating key involuntary functions such as heart rate, blood pressure, and respiratory activity across different stages of sleep.

Noting the segments of your nervous system

Your ANS influences your sleep and alternates between two states: the sympathetic and parasympathetic branches of the ANS, as shown in Figure 4-1:

>> **The *sympathetic* nervous system,** often called the fight-or-flight system, is more active during the day when you are awake and alert. It controls your body's response to acute stress, including various body functions by increasing

- Heart and respiratory rates
- Blood pressure
- Dilation of pupils

It is also responsible for decreases in digestion, salivation, and urination.

>> **The *parasympathetic* system,** which is associated with relaxation and recovery, dominates when you sleep. This shift in dominance between systems puts the parasympathetic system in charge of increasing digestion, salivation, and urination, and decreasing

- Heart and respiratory rates
- Blood pressure
- Dilation of pupils

These changes to body functions promote deep, restorative sleep.

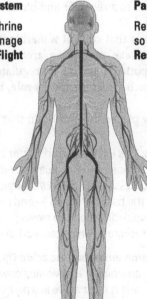

Autonomic Nervous System

Sympathetic nervous system

Releases norepinephrine and epinephrine to manage
Fight or Flight

Increases
- Heart rate
- Respiratory rate
- Blood pressure
- Pupil dilation

Decreases
- Salivation
- Digestion
- Urination

Parasympathetic nervous system

Releases acetylcholine so that you can
Rest and Digest

Increases
- Salivation
- Digestion
- Urination

Decreases
- Heart rate
- Respiratory rate
- Blood pressure
- Pupil dilation

FIGURE 4-1:
The sympathetic and parasympathetic segments of the ANS.

REMEMBER

Your ANS balances various physiological systems during different stages of sleep by releasing *neurotransmitters* — norepinephrine and epinephrine when the sympathetic system is active, and acetylcholine when the parasympathetic system takes over.

Enter the neurotransmitters and non-neurotransmitter substances

The nervous system communicates through chemical messengers called *neurotransmitters*. Several neurotransmitters work in harmony to regulate both NREM and REM sleep, which are two fundamental stages of sleep that offer different benefits to your brain and body. (See Chapter 2 for a discussion of these two sleep states/stages.) You can examine the interplay between the nervous system and your sleep architecture by exploring how different neurotransmitters regulate transitions between wakefulness and sleep and between NREM and REM. Also important to note is that these neurotransmitters typically bind to receptors in the central nervous system to generate a response. A table in Appendix A lists certain medications or substances that can serve as agonists (which bind to a receptor and produce an effect, often mimicking the actions of neurotransmitters) or antagonists (which bind to a receptor and block the action of an agonist).

The brain regions that control wakefulness and sleep each rely on specific neurotransmitters, wake-promoting areas in the brainstem, and sleep-promoting areas in the hypothalamus to help regulate deep, restorative sleep. For a detailed breakdown of each structure and its role, refer to the full table in Appendix A.

Some of the key players in your brain that regulate sleep include

>> **Adenosine:** This inhibitory transmitter affects several brain systems, including those nuclei involved in wakefulness. Adenosine inhibits systems associated with wakefulness — including *cholinergic* (which relate to acetylcholine) neurons in the basal forebrain — and promotes sleep and slow brain wave activity. Sleep deprivation can elevate adenosine, and caffeine can block adenosine receptors, which can lead to wakefulness.

>> **GABA (gamma-aminobutyric acid):** This neurotransmitter helps induce sleep by acting as an inhibitor and slowing down brain activity. GABA is essential for NREM sleep and is most active in a part of your brain called the *hypothalamus* — which also produces hormones that control some bodily functions — and specifically in the ventrolateral preoptic area (VLPO). *Neurons* (nerve cells that are part of your nervous system and use chemical and electrical signals to transmit information throughout your body) in the VLPO release GABA rapidly during sleep, especially in the deeper stages of NREM sleep. This activity helps shut down areas of the brain that keep you awake.

>> **Galanin:** This inhibitory neuropeptide works alongside GABA in promoting NREM sleep. Together, they suppress wake-promoting areas in the brain, which allows your brain to sleep.

>> **Glycine:** Like GABA, glycine also plays a role in suppressing wakefulness. It acts primarily in the *medulla*, which is part of the brainstem, and helps initiate and maintain NREM sleep.

Several neurotransmitters keep you alert and active during the day and shift the body between sleep stages. These chemicals are more active when you are awake and less active during sleep:

>> **Serotonin:** Found in the *raphe nuclei* (a cluster of neurons) in the brainstem, serotonin affects both sleep and wake regulation, although its role is complex and still under study. Serotonin tends to increase wakefulness, especially during the transitions out of sleep.

>> **Dopamine:** This neurotransmitter is essential for alertness and is most active during wakefulness and REM sleep. Reduced dopamine levels lead to decreased wakefulness and make it harder for you to stay alert.

>> **Histamine:** Produced by neurons in the hypothalamus, histamine keeps you awake. When histamine levels are high, they promote wakefulness. You may recognize the term *antihistamines* (medications that block histamine) and know that taking such a drug can induce drowsiness.

>> **Orexin (hypocretin):** A powerful neurotransmitter produced in the hypothalamus, orexin stabilizes wakefulness and prevents sudden transitions to sleep. People with narcolepsy often have low levels of orexin, which can lead to excessive sleepiness and disrupted sleep.

Other non–neurotransmitter substances that are important in sleep–wake regulation include

>> **Cytokines:** These proteins, such as *tumor necrosis factor-α* (TNF-α) and *interleukin-1β* (IL-1β), act as chemical messengers in the body's immune system. They can promote sleep and enhance slow-wave activity during sleep. If medications, such as those that treat cancer, block the cytokines, sleep is disrupted.

>> **Growth hormone-releasing hormone (GHRH):** This hormone is secreted by the hypothalamus and stimulates release of growth hormone by the pituitary. GHRH is important in NREM sleep regulation and specifically promotes NREM sleep.

>> **Melatonin:** This hormone receives various mentions in this book, but I want to emphasize its critical importance here.

REMEMBER

Melatonin is synthesized in the pineal gland from serotonin and has various effects related to sleep. Its synthesis and secretion are regulated by the *suprachiasmatic nucleus* (SCN, a cluster of neurons in your brain's hypothalamus; see the section "Checking the Circadian Clock and Chronobiology" later in the chapter for more) and suppressed by light. Melatonin also can promote dilation of blood vessels that can result in drops in body temperature. In this way, melatonin may consolidate and increase total sleep time, in addition to having impact on the timing of sleep and on circadian sleep-wake rhythms.

>> **Nitric oxide:** This signaling molecule is important in the regulation of NREM sleep and is produced in the basal forebrain and part of the hypothalamus.

>> **Prostaglandin-D$_2$:** This hormone-like compound activates a center in the preoptic area of the hypothalamus that promotes both NREM and REM sleep.

WARNING

Stress, poor diet, or certain medications can disrupt how these neurotransmitters and non-neurotransmitter substances work and, as a result, impact the quality of your sleep.

You can find a comprehensive list of naturally-occurring substances that affect sleep and wakefulness in Appendix A.

How sleeping pills and wake-promoting compounds affect the brain

When it comes to treating insomnia, the evolution of sleeping pills has been quite a journey.

WARNING

Sleeping pills and wake-promoting compounds, like any over-the-counter (OTC) or prescription medication, can have adverse or side effects, including dependence and *tolerance* (in which the body gets used to a drug after repeated use and requires higher doses to achieve the same effect). And so, discussing (with your physician) a compound's indications, adverse effects, and interactions with other medications is critically important before you take these or any medication.

If you take hypnotic medications for a long time (weeks, months, or even years), be aware that whenever you decide to stop taking the medications, you can expect insomnia to return for a few nights until the natural sleep-wake rhythm returns. You must expect this brief return to insomnia; it's important to recognize because, otherwise, you may be convinced that you have to take the medication in order to sleep.

Ideally, you should have your withdrawal from sleep medications supervised and coordinated with support from a sleep medicine specialist, who will usually recommend a gradual tapering off of these medications according to a schedule. Studies show that best outcomes occur for longest times with widely available cognitive behavioral treatments (CBT-I) for insomnia.

The main classes of sleeping pills at a glance

Here's a rundown of the main classes of sleep-promoting medications and how they work:

>> **First-generation — barbiturates:** These early sleep medications work by enhancing a brain chemical called gamma-aminobutyric acid (GABA), specifically at the $GABA_A$ receptor in the brain. Barbiturates are effective for inducing sleep, but they come with high risks — including dependence and respiratory depression — so they've mostly been replaced by safer options.

>> **Second-generation — benzodiazepines:** Developed as a safer alternative to barbiturates, benzodiazepines (such as diazepam, estazolam, flurazepam, lorazepam, quazepam, temazepam, and triazolam) also work by activating $GABA_A$ receptor. Benzodiazepines are generally safer, but they still have some risks, which include potential for abuse, side effects (such as respiratory depression), and *rebound insomnia* (insomnia that worsens after stopping the medication).

>> **Third-generation — non-benzodiazepine hypnotics:** These medications (including zolpidem, zaleplon, and eszopiclone) became popular in the 1980s for their lower risk of dependence and fewer side effects (when compared to benzodiazepines). These medications, which also activate GABA, are categorized based on the duration of their action:

- *Short-acting hypnotics (like zolpidem* and *zaleplon)* have short half-lives of one hour and one to three hours, respectively, making them suitable for people who have trouble falling asleep but need to avoid next-day grogginess.

- *Longer-acting hypnotics (like extended-release zolpidem, or zolpidem CR, and eszopiclone)* have longer half-lives of around six hours (for eszopiclone) and are prescribed for patients who struggle with either staying asleep or both falling and staying asleep.

- *Antidepressants like doxepin* can work as a sleep aid by blocking histamine (H1) receptors that are found in many cells and tissues of the body. Doxepin is known for increasing total sleep time and reducing *wake after sleep onset* (WASO), which means that it helps you stay asleep longer.

- *A short-acting hypnotic, ramelteon, works like melatonin.* It has a half-life of about one to three hours and binds to melatonin receptors (MT1 and

MT2). This medication is not associated with dependence, abuse, or rebound insomnia when stopped, which makes it a safer choice for some sleep medication users.

>> **New kids on the block — DORAs:** These dual orexin receptor antagonists (DORAs), such as daridorexant, lemborexant, and suvorexant, work differently from GABA-targeting medications. They promote sleep by blocking the brain's wakefulness signals at both orexin receptors (OX1 and OX2) in the brain and peripheral areas of the body. DORAs are effective for people who need help with falling and/or staying asleep, and they generally don't cause tolerance, withdrawal symptoms, or rebound insomnia when stopped.

Over-the-counter (OTC) sleep aids

If you prefer to take OTC drugs, or need alternatives to traditional sleep medications, you have options:

>> **Antihistamines:** Some OTC antihistamines — such as diphenhydramine, doxylamine, and promethazine — are sometimes used as sleep aids because of their sedating effects. However, they have relatively long half-lives (3.4 to 9.2 hours for diphenhydramine, 10 hours for doxylamine, and 12–15 hours for promethazine), which can lead to next-day grogginess or *hangover* effects. In older adults, these medications may also cause adverse neurocognitive effects, so caution is advised.

>> **Melatonin:** OTC melatonin has a short half-life of about 20–30 minutes, so it helps people fall asleep faster by reducing *sleep latency* (the time it takes to fall asleep). However, melatonin has limited effects on sleep structure, so it may not enhance either deep NREM sleep (N3) or REM sleep stages. Melatonin is especially useful for people dealing with circadian rhythm disorders (such as jet lag or shift work).

REMEMBER

Each type of sleep aid has its own benefits and potential downsides. Talk to your doctor to find the option that's best for your sleep needs and lifestyle.

To read a detailed table covering common prescription sleeping pills that are FDA-approved for the treatment of insomnia, their drug class, and how they work, turn to Appendix A.

Understanding wake-promoting medications and substances

If you struggle with excessive daytime sleepiness (EDS), several types of medications exist that may help. People with conditions such as narcolepsy or idiopathic hypersomnia often use them.

Each one of these medications works in a unique way to keep you alert:

» **Modafinil and armodafinil:** These medications treat EDS but provide a more gradual onset and offset of sleep than do stimulant-like medications. This trait reduces the risk of an abrupt *crash* to a state of sleepiness. However, they have somewhat milder stimulating effects compared to amphetamines.

» **Pitolisant:** This drug is approved for treating EDS and cataplexy (a sudden loss of muscle tone) in people with narcolepsy. Pitolisant works by raising histamine levels in the brain. It also seems to boost other wake-promoting neurotransmitters, such as acetylcholine, dopamine, and norepinephrine.

» **Sodium oxybate:** This drug is used to treat both the EDS and cataplexy in people with narcolepsy — and a low-sodium version that combines calcium, magnesium, and potassium salts — also treats these conditions, as well as EDS in those with idiopathic hypersomnia. Sodium oxybate binds to $GABA_B$ receptors in the brain to promote deep, consolidated nighttime sleep, which reduces EDS during the day. Typically, sodium oxybate is taken twice per night, although a once-nightly version is also available.

» **Solriamfetol:** This medication treats EDS for people with obstructive sleep apnea or narcolepsy by increasing dopamine and norepinephrine levels in the brain, which helps you stay awake longer.

» **Stimulants and stimulant-like medications:** Stimulant medications such as amphetamine and methylphenidate (Ritalin) are common EDS treatments. These drugs can be quite effective, but they come with some potential downsides. For example, they can be habit-forming and may cause a tendency toward misuse or abuse. Their effects also tend to start and stop abruptly, which can sometimes cause a sudden *crash* to drowsiness or even *sleep attacks* (in which sleepiness hits quickly and without warning).

To see a detailed list covering common prescription wake–promoting compounds or stimulants, their drug class, their FDA-approved indication for sleep-wake problems or disorders, and how they work, turn to Appendix A.

A note about caffeine

People worldwide use caffeine widely in beverages and OTC supplements to boost alertness. It works by blocking adenosine receptors in the brain, which enhances wakefulness. While caffeine is safe and effective, it isn't strong enough on its own to counteract the severe EDS that is a symptom of narcolepsy or idiopathic hypersomnia, so people often use it as a supplement to medications prescribed for these sleep disorders.

Regulating Wake-Sleep and NREM versus REM sleep

To stay awake, your brain relies on a group of its connected regions called the *ascending reticular activating system (ARAS)*. This system, which includes several important nuclei, is like the brain's wakefulness network. See Figure 4-2. In the ARAS, you find

>> **Basal forebrain:** This area receives signals from the brainstem and hypothalamus. It plays a big role in activating the cortex during both wakefulness and REM sleep.

>> **Laterodorsal tegmental (LDT) and pedunculopontine tegmental (PPT) nuclei:** These brainstem regions promote both wakefulness and REM sleep.

>> **Locus coeruleus (LC), raphe nuclei (RN), and tuberomammillary nucleus (TMN):** These key areas in the ARAS work together to keep you alert and active.

>> **Ventral tegmental area (VTA) and substantia nigra (SN):** These regions support wakefulness and prevent sleep by managing emotional and motor behaviors, which help you stay engaged and responsive.

To keep you awake, the ARAS uses a combination of neurotransmitters, including acetylcholine, dopamine, epinephrine, and norepinephrine. You can find out more about neurotransmitters in the section "Enter the neurotransmitters and non-neurotransmitter substances" earlier in the chapter.

How the brain decides between sleep and wakefulness

When it's time for you to sleep, another part of your brain takes charge. The *ventrolateral preoptic (VLPO) nucleus* works as your brain's sleep switch, mainly by releasing GABA (an inhibiting neurotransmitter). The VLPO nucleus and the ARAS work in opposition — a relationship called the *flip-flop sleep switch model*, first proposed by Dr. Clifford Saper and his colleagues at Harvard in the 2000s. Refer to Figure 4-3 for the relevant brain regions and nuclei.

When the ARAS is more active than the VLPO, you stay awake. When the VLPO is more active than the ARAS, you fall asleep. This flip-flop switch changes depending on which area in your brain is more active, giving you a clear-cut outcome of either wakefulness or sleep.

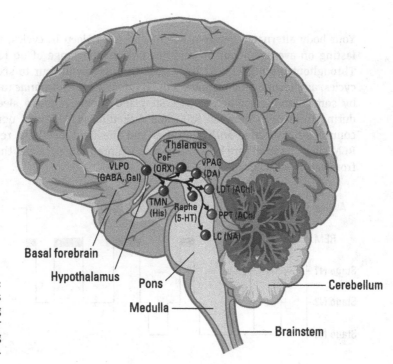

FIGURE 4-2: The brain's ascending reticular activating system (ARAS).

And the *orexin (hypocretin) neurons* in the hypothalamus add an extra layer to this sleep-switch process. The VLPO usually inhibits orexin neurons to promote sleep. However, when the ARAS is active, the VLPO stops suppressing the orexin neurons, allowing them to boost the ARAS even further, leading to sustained wakefulness.

The brain's role during sleep stages

Your sleep is divided into two major types: non-rapid eye movement (NREM) sleep and rapid eye movement (REM) sleep. These stages of sleep serve different functions in your body and are regulated by particular parts of your brain, specifically

>> **NREM sleep:** Consists of three stages, each one progressively deeper than the last. (See Chapter 2 for a description of these three stages.) During this stage, your body focuses on repair and recovery. Blood pressure lowers, muscles relax (compared to their state in wakefulness), and tissue growth occurs. Also during NREM sleep, your brain consolidates memories and processes information.

>> **REM sleep:** Associated with dreaming and memory consolidation, this is a lighter stage of sleep in which your brain is very active. During REM, your voluntary muscles are in a state of paralysis (to prevent you from acting out your dreams).

Your body alternates between NREM and REM sleep in cycles, with each cycle lasting on average about 90 minutes (within the range of 60 to 120 minutes). Throughout the night, your body goes through about four to six of these sleep cycles, as shown by the histogram in Figure 4-3. *Norepinephrine* (a chemical made by some nerve cells in the adrenal gland) helps regulate sleep, particularly during transitions between REM and wakefulness. Although norepinephrine is commonly associated with alertness and the fight-or-flight response, during REM sleep, its levels are kept low to help maintain the paralysis that prevents you from acting out your dreams.

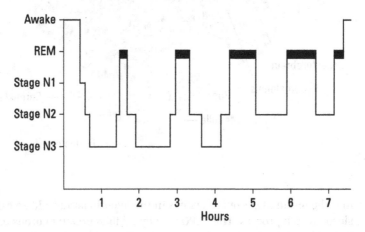

FIGURE 4-3:
A sleep cycle histogram.

Various brain areas and nuclei are involved with the divisions of sleep:

>> **For NREM sleep** (the deep, restful stage of sleep) to occur, a part of your brain called the *preoptic anterior hypothalamus (POAH)* plays a crucial role. This area, located just above where the optic nerves meet, contains two key groups of neurons: the VLPO nucleus and the *median preoptic nucleus (MnPN)*. As you start to fall asleep, neurons within the brainstem's wake-promoting systems begin to slow down. The VLPO, in particular, releases the inhibiting neurotransmitter GABA to help switch your brain into sleep mode.

>> **For REM sleep,** the stage associated with dreaming, your body relies on the *laterodorsal tegmental (LDT)* and *pedunculopontine tegmental (PPT) nuclei*. These areas use acetylcholine (also a neurotransmitter) to create the unique features of REM sleep, including rapid eye movements, increased brain activity, and temporary muscle paralysis. During REM sleep, GABA-containing neurons in the basal forebrain send signals to the hypothalamus and brainstem, suppressing the wake-promoting neurons and helping you stay in this sleep stage.

REMEMBER

Both NREM and REM sleep are critical for physical and mental health. The regulation of sleep is delicate; disruptions in either state can lead to sleep disorders or poor sleep quality. For example, disruptions in neurotransmitter levels or brain regions responsible for sleep regulation can lead to sleep disorders such as *insomnia* (when you can't sleep) or conditions like *narcolepsy* (in which REM sleep intrudes unexpectedly into wakefulness).

Adjusting your sleep habits to maintain sleep-stage balance

TIP

To help your neurotransmitters (see the preceding section) fine-tune your NREM and REM sleep, you can

>> **Minimize disruptions:** Limit exposure to blue light (from devices such as smartphones and computers) before bed because blue light interferes with production of the hormone melatonin. And melatonin is critical for maintaining your circadian rhythm and promoting REM sleep. (See the section "Endocrine system" later in the chapter for more information about melatonin.)

>> **Regulate stress:** Elevated levels of the neurotransmitter norepinephrine — which may result from chronic stress — can impair your ability to transition smoothly into REM sleep because it keeps your body on alert. Practices such as deep breathing or meditation before bed can help reduce stress hormones and allow neurotransmitters like GABA to do their job in promoting deeper sleep.

>> **Keep a regular schedule:** Going to bed and waking up at the same time each day helps stabilize your sleep-wake cycle, enabling neurotransmitters such as serotonin to facilitate a smoother transition into sleep stages.

TECHNICAL STUFF

PARASOMNIAS AND SLEEP STAGES

Parasomnias are abnormal behaviors or experiences that occur during sleep, often reflecting a mixture of wake, NREM, and REM states. That is, parasomnia disorders seem to involve a dissociation of brain activity — parts of the brain remain in a sleep state while other parts awaken. For example, during sleepwalking episodes, motor functions become active while the cognitive centers remain largely asleep, leading to complex behaviors performed without conscious awareness.

(continued)

(continued)

Additionally, research suggests that parasomnias — like REM sleep behavior disorder (RBD) — may have a neurological basis because they often link to disruptions in the brainstem, specifically to areas that regulate REM sleep. And because these regions also participate in maintaining circadian rhythms, any dysregulation there can contribute to parasomnia episodes.

Parasomnias can occur in both main stages of sleep:

- **NREM parasomnias** typically occur during the deeper stages of NREM sleep, often during the first third of the night. Examples include sleepwalking and sleep (night) terrors. These parasomnias often link with fragmented sleep and a phenomenon called cyclic alternating pattern (CAP), which represents periods of instability in NREM sleep, as seen through EEG measurements.

- **REM sleep parasomnias,** such as RBD, occur when muscle paralysis fails during REM sleep, allowing individuals to act out their dreams. Norepinephrine plays a key role in regulating these transitions into and out of REM sleep. When this system is disrupted, individuals may experience vivid and sometimes violent dream enactment behaviors. Additionally, research has shown that parasomnias in REM sleep involve increased brain activity in specific regions, often linked to emotional processing and movement.

Both types of parasomnias can follow from internal and external factors that fragment sleep, such as obstructive sleep apnea, bright light exposure at night, shift work or jet lag, or noise disturbances. These triggers disrupt the brain's ability to maintain stable sleep stages, increasing the risk of parasomnias occurring. (See Chapter 8 for a more detailed discussion of parasomnia disorders.)

Exploring How Sleep Affects Your Body

Sleep doesn't just give your mind a chance to recharge; it also plays a crucial role in maintaining your physical health. During sleep, your body works to repair tissues, regulate vital systems, and process essential hormones. Every system in your body — from the respiratory to the cardiovascular — relies on adequate sleep to function properly. Without the right amount and quality of rest, both the body and mind are affected, which can lead to various negative health and well-being consequences.

Sleep and the respiratory system

Your respiratory system doesn't take a break while you sleep. In fact, it works closely with your brain to ensure that you maintain steady and efficient breathing patterns during rest.

REMEMBER

During certain stages of sleep, particularly NREM sleep, your breathing slows down significantly, and the muscles that control your airways relax. From wakefulness to NREM (N1 and N2) stages, some respiratory instability exists because the breathing switches from any conscious control to an automatic mechanism. When deeper NREM (N3) sleep occurs, you experience a more regular breathing pattern. (See Chapter 8 for information about sleep apnea.)

During REM sleep, breathing becomes more irregular and results in a mix of patterns with rapid shallow breaths and pauses in between them. These changes are normal and part of your body's natural sleep cycle. However, if you have a condition that affects your airways or lung function — such as asthma or chronic obstructive pulmonary disease (COPD) — these respiratory changes during sleep can exacerbate your symptoms and lead to disruptions in sleep quality. Additionally, for those patients who have obstructive sleep apnea (OSA), the instability of the respiratory system during REM sleep results in worsening of their abnormal breathing during this sleep state characterized by more frequent breathing pauses and drops in oxygen.

TIP

If you experience difficulty breathing during sleep, speak with a healthcare provider. Many sleep-related respiratory conditions are treatable or manageable with lifestyle changes or medical interventions.

TECHNICAL STUFF

OBSTRUCTIVE SLEEP APNEA (OSA)

Obstructive sleep apnea (OSA) doesn't just affect your breathing; it also frequently interrupts your sleep throughout the night, causing fragmented sleep and disrupting the natural transitions between NREM and REM stages. This disruption can throw your body out of sync, leading to broader issues with sleep quality and overall health. Chapter 8 has more details on OSA.

The repeated awakenings and alterations in the release of key neurotransmitters and hormones caused by OSA prevent your body from cycling through the normal stages of sleep in a smooth, orderly way. For example,

- Each time your airway collapses and you wake up, it triggers an increase in sympathetic nervous system activity with norepinephrine and epinephrine — your body's

(continued)

(continued)

fight-or-flight response. This stress response raises your blood pressure and heart rate, counteracting the parasympathetic "rest-and-digest" processes with acetylcholine that help restore and repair your body during sleep.

- The release of melatonin — your body's sleep-promoting hormone — can be affected by OSA. Melatonin normally rises at night to signal your brain that it's time to sleep, but frequent OSA-related awakenings can throw off this hormonal rhythm and make falling and staying asleep more difficult.

- Sleep fragmentation associated with OSA affects the body's ability to properly regulate cortisol — a stress hormone. Elevated cortisol levels can perpetuate sleep disruptions and create a cycle of poor sleep quality and daytime fatigue.

- In a child with OSA, the abnormal breathing events that fragment sleep can alter the secretion pattern of growth hormone. This, in turn, can cause the child to have delayed growth and make them fall off the normal age-related growth curve for height and weight.

- Women who enter menopause may develop OSA or have it worsened, presumably by the reduction of estrogen and progesterone that occurs during menopause. Researchers believe that these hormones may protect the upper airway in premenopausal women, and when menopause happens, this protection diminishes. This results in the prevalence of OSA in postmenopausal women approaching that of men.

OSA also has a significant effect on the cardiovascular system, and the risk for developing hypertension increases with OSA severity. Patients who have OSA have a greater risk for conditions such as *cardiac arrhythmias* (including atrial fibrillation) and heart failure.

Sleep and the cardiovascular system

Your cardiovascular system relies heavily on the restorative functions of sleep to maintain heart health. For example,

>> **During deep stages of NREM sleep,** your heart rate slows and your blood pressure lowers to allow your heart to rest and recover. This nightly relaxation phase is crucial for long-term heart health because it gives your cardiovascular system a break from the constant demands of wakefulness.

>> **During REM sleep** (this stage is associated with brain activity comparable to that of wakefulness), your heart rate and blood pressure can fluctuate more, simulating the variations you experience when you're awake. These fluctuations are normal and necessary for maintaining the flexibility and responsiveness of your cardiovascular system. However, when sleep is disrupted, these natural processes become dysregulated, and sleep doesn't get to do the work it needs to do.

WARNING

If you experience fragmented sleep, your body doesn't spend enough time in the deep NREM sleep stages that are essential for your health. Chronic sleep deprivation or poor-quality sleep can lead to increased risk of cardiovascular problems, including

>> **Increased hypertension risk:** Sleep deprivation elevates blood pressure and increases the risk of heart disease and stroke.

WARNING

If you have habitual short sleep — that is, if you average less than six hours of sleep on weekdays — and try *catch-up sleep* (in which you try to recover your sleep periodically after bouts of short sleep), you won't significantly reduce your blood pressure.

>> **Increased cardiovascular disease:** Shortened sleep is associated with increased cardiovascular disease and elevated mortality.

>> **Heightened stress response:** Fragmented sleep leads to higher cortisol levels, which puts more stress on your heart.

>> **Disrupted metabolism:** Lack of sleep affects how your body processes glucose and manages appetite, contributing to weight gain and increasing the risk of heart disease.

Sleep and other body systems

Sleep plays a vital role in regulating many of your body's systems, beyond just the heart and lungs. The digestive, endocrine, and thermoregulatory systems all experience significant changes while you sleep. Here's a look at how these systems interact with your sleep and circadian sleep-wake mechanisms.

Digestive system

Your digestive system follows a circadian sleep-wake rhythm that impacts how your body processes food throughout the day and night. For example, gastric acid secretion follows a strong circadian pattern, peaking in the early morning hours between midnight and 2 a.m. but does not appear tied to a specific sleep stage. This surge is sometimes referred to as *nocturnal acid breakthrough*.

Although the relationship between sleep stages and acid secretion is not well established, evidence suggests that *gastric motility* — the movement of food through your digestive system — varies significantly during sleep. Esophageal activity decreases, and the *upper esophageal sphincter* (UES) relaxes. The UES is a ring of muscle located at the top of the esophagus, where the throat meets the esophagus, and it functions to

>> **Open and allow food and liquid to pass into the esophagus** while preventing air from entering the esophagus and stomach during breathing.

>> **Prevent food and stomach acids from traveling back up the esophagus,** reducing the risk of reflux. Relaxation of the UES can increase the likelihood of acid reflux, particularly if you eat late or consume large meals before bed.

Many episodes of *gastroesophageal reflux* (GER, in which stomach contents move into the esophagus) occur just before waking and demonstrate how digestive activity is closely linked to your circadian rhythm. During REM sleep, your digestion is generally more active, and as you approach waking, the digestive system reactivates. When you're awake, GER normally occurs after eating (usually within an hour); during sleep, it primarily occurs during the lighter stages of sleep and when awakening from sleep.

TIP

If you're prone to heartburn or acid reflux, try eating smaller, lighter meals in the evening. Avoid lying down right after eating, because doing so can exacerbate reflux, especially during the relaxed state of sleep. Keeping your digestive system calm before bed will help reduce digestive discomfort.

Aside from GER, sleep also impacts other areas of your digestive health, including

>> **The rest-and-digest functions** of the parasympathetic nervous system (described in the section "Noting the segments of your nervous system" earlier in the chapter) are more active during sleep, which allows your body to process and store nutrients more effectively.

>> **The motor activity of the small bowel** involves a wave of contractions that begins in the stomach and proceeds through the rest of the GI tract. Interestingly, when food is not in the stomach, the wave of contractions has a period of about 90 minutes, which is similar to the normal NREM-REM sleep cycle.

>> **The motor activity of the colon** is usually inhibited during sleep, but upon awakening from sleep (such as when you get up in the morning), the situation changes. The colon activity at this time produces strong contractions of the colon that are frequently associated with an urge to defecate.

WARNING

Chronic sleep deprivation (which I discuss in Chapter 3) can lead to disruptions in the *gut-brain axis* that connects the brain and the gastrointestinal tract, resulting in digestive issues such as bloating, constipation, and even inflammatory responses.

To support healthy digestion, maintain a regular sleep schedule and practice relaxation techniques before bed, such as deep breathing or meditation. These activities engage your parasympathetic nervous system, promoting better digestion and reducing gastrointestinal discomfort

Musculoskeletal system

One of sleep's most important functions is muscle recovery and tissue repair. During deep NREM sleep, the body secretes growth hormone, which aids in muscle growth, tissue recovery, and healing from injuries. This stage is particularly critical for athletes or those recovering from physical stress. Lack of sleep can lead to muscle fatigue and slower recovery times. On the other hand, REM sleep, which comes later in the cycle, plays a role in brain functions such as emotional regulation but also inhibits muscle tone by relaxing the body's skeletal muscles (aside from small muscle twitches).

REMEMBER

Consistent, high-quality sleep supports muscle recovery and tissue repair. Whether you're an athlete or just want to recover from daily physical strain, your body needs those deep sleep cycles to restore and rebuild. Make sleep a priority just like you would your exercise routine.

Endocrine system

Your endocrine system links closely with your sleep-wake cycle by releasing hormones at certain times. As darkness falls, your body produces melatonin, a hormone that signals your brain it's time to sleep. As morning approaches, your cortisol levels begin to rise, helping you wake up and feel alert. Disruptions to your sleep or circadian sleep-wake rhythm can throw these hormone levels out of sync.

Sleep has a significant influence on your body's hormone levels, particularly through the *hypothalamus-pituitary-adrenal (HPA) axis*, a neuroendocrine system that regulates the body's stress response and includes the hypothalamus, pituitary glands, and adrenal glands. This system governs hormones such as cortisol and *adrenocorticotropic hormone (ACTH)*, which affect nearly every organ and tissue in your body. Hormones from the HPA follow a distinct pattern during sleep — for example,

>> **Growth hormone levels,** as secreted from the pituitary gland, surge during slow-wave sleep, aiding in the repair and growth of tissues.

>> **Cortisol levels** are at their lowest during the first half of the night and then rise in the early morning hours as part of your body's preparation for wakefulness.

>> **Thyroid hormone levels** tend to decrease during sleep (but increase with sleep deprivation). An overactive thyroid (hyperthyroidism) and underactive thyroid (hypothyroidism) can result in difficulty falling and staying asleep, and hypothyroidism is also associated with excessive sleepiness.

>> **Renin levels** are important for kidney function; they tend to rise during NREM sleep and peak during REM sleep, which indicates that your body is regulating vital kidney functions even as you rest.

WARNING

Sleep also influences insulin sensitivity and glucose metabolism, meaning that disrupted or insufficient sleep can raise your risk of developing metabolic conditions such as diabetes. Research has shown that people who consistently sleep less than six hours a night have a higher risk of insulin resistance.

Thermoregulation

Your body temperature fluctuates on a circadian sleep-wake schedule, peaking around 9 p.m. Then it starts to drop, which facilitates sleep onset. Core body temperature reaches its lowest point in the early morning hours, around 5 a.m. During NREM sleep, your core body temperature drops, helping your body conserve energy and enabling restorative processes to take place. By the time you enter REM sleep, your body temperature begins to stabilize, and you remain in a near-thermoneutral state.

A drop in core body temperature is crucial for the onset of sleep and is managed by a complex process of *vasodilation*, where blood vessels in your skin widen to release heat. This process is regulated by melatonin, a hormone that is not only involved in sleep initiation but also plays a role in cooling your body for sleep.

However, during REM sleep, thermoregulation becomes less efficient. For instance, your body's ability to manage heat loss through the skin can be compromised, leading to unpredictable fluctuations in body temperature.

TIP

To optimize your sleep environment, aim to keep your bedroom temperature between 60- and 67-degrees Fahrenheit. A cooler room can help your body stay in its natural temperature-lowering state, allowing for deeper, more restorative sleep.

Immune system

During sleep, your body's immune system goes into high gear, producing and releasing proteins known as *cytokines* that help fight infection and inflammation. This immune response is why you often feel extra tired when you're sick — your body is trying to devote more resources to recovery.

Studies show that people who don't get enough sleep are more likely to get sick after being exposed to a virus, such as the common cold, and may also be slower to recover from illness. Adequate sleep is essential for a strong immune response. If you feel under the weather or are recovering from an illness, make sure to prioritize rest to give your body the best chance to heal.

Checking the Circadian Clock and Chronobiology

Circadian (a word derived from the Latin *circa diem*, which means "about a day") *rhythms* are the sequence of the body processes that correspond to an approximate 24-hour cycle. Your sleep–wake cycle is largely governed by two main biological processes that work together to control this cycle. Disruptions to either of these processes can lead to sleep issues:

>> **Process S** represents your body's homeostatic sleep drive, which accumulates the longer you're awake. (The word *homeostatic* describes the process by which living organisms maintain a steady internal environment.) And Process S governs the intensity of your sleep need, The more time you've spent awake, the greater your need for sleep becomes by nightfall. During sleep, the sleep drive dissipates, restoring your body's sleep-wake balance and preparing you for the next day.

>> **Process C,** on the other hand, refers to your circadian rhythm, which follows a roughly 24-hour cycle. This process is regulated by environmental cues such as light, temperature, and social cues (for example, work and family activities). It dictates when you feel alert during the day and when you get drowsy at night to help you maintain a consistent sleep schedule and ensure that sleep occurs at the right time.

At the center of Process C is the *suprachiasmatic nucleus (SCN)*, a cluster of neurons in your brain's hypothalamus located just above the optic chiasm, where the optic nerves cross. The SCN is highly sensitive to light exposure and functions as your body's master clock to regulate your sleep-wake cycle and other circadian rhythms. It responds to light signals, influencing the timing of your sleep and wake periods. The SCN also has an effect on the flip-flop sleep switch mechanism (see its description in the section "How the brain decides between sleep and wakefulness" earlier in the chapter). The SCN sends neuronal outputs to the ARAS and VLPO nuclei that, in turn, can regulate the timing of the switch between wakefulness and sleep.

The concept of Process S and Process C (as depicted in Figure 4-4) was originally proposed by pioneering sleep researcher Alexander Borbély and his team. Borbély is widely credited with developing the *two-process model of sleep regulation* in the late 1980s, which became a foundational framework for understanding how sleep pressure (Process S) and circadian sleep-wake rhythms (Process C) interact. His work underscored the importance of balancing sleep drive with circadian cues to achieve optimal sleep and wake patterns.

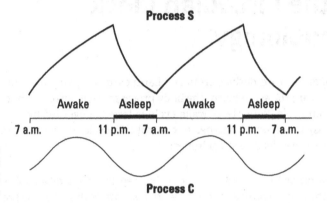

FIGURE 4-4:
Process S and
Process C
working together.

Genes that govern your circadian rhythm

A set of *clock genes* governs the SCN's functioning (see the preceding section) and drives the *expression* of proteins regulating the daily rhythm of these neurons (*expression*, in this case, refers to the process by which information in the genes is turned into functional proteins). Among the most significant are the *per* (period) and *cry* (cryptochrome) genes, which are essential to the circadian cycle. The expression of these genes generates rhythmic activity in the SCN, which in turn sends signals to the various parts of your brain that control the circadian patterns in physiology that occur in sleep and wakefulness.

Environmental cues: Light and zeitgebers

One of the most powerful influences on your circadian sleep-wake rhythm is light. When light hits your retina, it sends signals to the SCN, which can either advance or delay your sleep cycle. Specifically, exposure to light

>> **In the morning** can help phase-advance your sleep cycle, which allows you to wake up earlier

>> **In the evening** can phase-delay your cycle, which pushes your bedtime later

Even small amounts of light, such as 40 lux (similar to low room lighting), can have a significant effect on the SCN. Blue light, in particular, is potent, which is why many apps and devices now offer blue-light filtering and blocking options.

Besides light, other environmental factors known as *zeitgebers* (from the German for time-givers) can influence your circadian sleep-wake rhythm. These factors include temperature, clocks, physical activity (exercise), meal timing, and social interactions. Exercise, for instance, can also shift your sleep cycle depending on when you're active. For example, morning exercise can phase-advance your sleep cycle, making you sleepy earlier, while evening exercise may phase-delay it.

When individuals are isolated from zeitgebers (such as being in a dark cave), the individual can *free run*, meaning that the internal circadian sleep-wake rhythm fails to align with the 24-hour day and night cycle driven by the sun. Because individuals have a slightly longer internal circadian cycle of about 24.5–24.7 hours, the free run natural tendency is to want to sleep a little later and also awaken a little later during each successive circadian cycle. For individuals who aren't voluntarily isolated from zeitgebers, this situation is called a non-24-hour sleep-wake disorder (N24). This disorder is common in individuals who are blind as well as in some non-visually impaired individuals who may have dysfunction of their SCN.

Peripheral clocks

While the SCN is your body's central pacemaker for regulating circadian sleep-wake rhythms, you also have peripheral clocks located in tissues throughout your body. These clocks, although self-sustaining, rely on the SCN to stay synchronized. They regulate various metabolic functions — such as blood glucose levels during sleep — and prepare your body for the day ahead by mechanisms such as boosting cardiovascular function and increasing cortisol levels.

When the SCN becomes uncoupled from your peripheral clocks — such as in cases of starvation or shift work — the result can include metabolic issues and other health problems. For example, individuals who work night shifts are at higher risk for metabolic disorders, obesity, type 2 diabetes, and cardiovascular diseases due to the desynchronization of these peripheral clocks.

Cognitive and physical performance

The SCN influences your cognitive and physical performance throughout the day, most likely coupled with output from the *locus coeruleus* (LC), which promotes wakefulness and has been associated with attention, learning, memory, and higher-order cognitive functioning. Cognitive functions such as paying attention, problem-solving, and making memories tend to follow your circadian rhythm. They peak when your core body temperature is highest in the late afternoon.

Conversely, performance declines during the night, particularly when melatonin levels are at their peak and core body temperature is at its lowest. This condition explains why tasks that require complex problem-solving, focus, and hand-eye coordination are more difficult late at night, particularly for shift workers who operate outside the typical circadian sleep-wake rhythm.

IN THIS CHAPTER

» Exploring different theories on
why you dream

» Learning how to study and interpret
your dreams

» Understanding how psychological
and psychiatric disorders impact
your dreams

» Recognizing and controlling
your dreams

Chapter 5

Discovering Dreaming

Dreams have fascinated people for centuries, with some of the earliest recorded theories dating back to Aristotle. Over time, scientists and philosophers alike have speculated about the purpose of dreams — why people dream, what dreams mean, and how they might affect waking life. In this chapter, I explore those ideas and dive into modern scientific investigations that offer insight into what happens in your brain while you dream.

I also explain how psychology and psychiatry influence modern society's understanding of dreams, particularly in relation to anxiety, PTSD, and depression. Additionally, I cover the fascinating phenomenon of lucid dreaming in which you can not only recognize that you're dreaming, but also perhaps control your dreams while they're happening.

Theorizing on the Purpose of Dreams

Aristotle made some of the earliest commentaries about dreaming. He disseminated three main essays on sleep: *On Sleep and Waking*, *On Dreams*, and *On Divination in Sleep*. In these essays, Aristotle explored his theories about dreams, questioning whether dreams could be interpreted or used to predict future events.

He argued that dreams weren't messages from the gods but rather the result of physical processes happening within the body. Aristotle even suggested that when dreams seem predictive, the related situation was likely just a coincidence.

Since Aristotle's time, specialists have explored other theories and conducted scientific investigations into dreaming. In particular, they ramped up in the 1950s with the discovery of REM sleep (to read more on the discovery of REM sleep, turn to Chapter 2). These theories suggest

REMEMBER

>> **You dream as part of your learning and memory consolidation process, where your brain replays and processes emotionally charged daytime experiences.** Neuroimaging studies even show a relationship between dreaming and recalling past experiences or imagining future scenarios. These studies suggest that dreams enhance learning and often incorporate specific elements of tasks you learn before sleeping.

>> **Dreams help you contextualize waking experiences and prepare for future events by making connections in the safe environment of a dream.** Emotional waking experiences tend to show up in your dreams — more frequently than neutral ones — and can help you emotionally adapt to intense experiences in real life.

>> **Dreaming might provide people with realistic simulation of threats (a hypothesis known as the *threat simulation theory*).** If you experience and react to threats in dreams — for example, being chased or facing a natural disaster — this experience might enhance your chances of survival if you encounter such threats in waking life. That is, successfully managing a threat during dreams may help you appropriately react if you come upon that threat in real life.

But one challenge to this theory is that a lot of dream content has positive emotions, which indicates that this theory captures only a portion of dreams.

>> **Dreaming simulates various types of social interactions, which might enhance your social skills (a hypothesis known as the *social simulation theory*).** Many dreams involve social interactions, and many people report having these interactions more frequently in dreams than they do in waking experiences. Social interactions in dreams tend to be more realistic and emotionally relevant when compared to other dream content that features solitary situations, such as dreaming of taking a hike or working alone in your home. Because humans' survival depends on successful social interaction, these simulated interactions could be an adaptive advantage in waking life.

REMEMBER

So far, no evidence exists that dreams serve an evolutionary function, though REM sleep (during which most dreams occur) also happens in non-human species. In the end, dreams may just be behavioral events that don't correspond to any vital function.

Studying and Interpreting Dreams

An early method of studying dreams involved researchers collecting anecdotal reports from individuals about their dreams. Over time, they developed more scientific and structured frameworks. For example, researchers instructed participants to

>> **Write down their dream reports upon waking,** either in the morning or during nighttime awakenings. Participants recorded these reports over several days or weeks.

>> **Answer specific questions** about the themes or types of dreams, such as whether they were regular dreams or nightmares.

>> **Compare dream imagery** to photographs with varying degrees of brightness or color.

In the 1960s and 1970s, researchers refined their classifications of dream content by using tools such as scales and questionnaires to complement the dream reports. In more recent years, they employed sophisticated algorithms — including some artificial intelligence (AI) models — to systematically analyze dream content.

Detecting brain activity

To understand how your brain behaves during dreams, scientists use advanced imaging techniques such as *functional magnetic resonance imaging* (fMRI) and *positron emission tomography* (PET). These tools enable the imaging of various structures in the brain and track changes in blood flow and metabolism, respectively. Having these data allow researchers to compare brain activity during wakefulness, REM sleep, and slow-wave sleep.

Studies show that during REM sleep, blood flow increases to associative visual areas and limbic regions, which are the areas of the brain involved in emotion. This explains why dreams can be so visually rich and emotionally charged. On the other hand, the frontal areas of your brain, which are responsible for consciousness and decision-making, show reduced activity during REM sleep. This decrease in frontal brain activity is likely why you have less awareness or control during most dreams.

Researchers also apply *electroencephalogram* (EEG) electrodes overlying all of the major brain areas of patients in addition to those EEG electrodes applied during typical polysomnography or sleep studies (see Chapter 10 for more information). The goal is to understand brain waves that occur while the patient is dreaming versus those that exist when they're not dreaming. In these EEG studies, they've found key patterns related to brain wave frequencies, which they measured in hertz (Hz), or cycles per second:

>> **Slow-wave activity (0.5 to 4 hertz)** is characteristic of deep sleep and is negatively associated with dreaming in both NREM (non-REM) and REM sleep. In other words, if you have more slow-wave activity, you're less likely to dream. Researchers are exploring whether this distinction could serve as a *biomarker* (a measurable biological characteristic that may indicate a normal versus abnormal process) for dreaming — or the absence of dreaming — in the future.

>> **Sleep spindles (12 to 14 hertz)** are more frequent in the posterior regions of the brain during NREM sleep. Faster spindles during the night may be associated with more vivid dream recall.

Researchers have observed that slow-wave activity may affect your ability to recall dreams. You're more likely to report dreams when sleep spindles show a higher frequency in the posterior regions of the brain, known as the *posterior hot zone*, which includes portions of the occipital lobe and other posterior brain regions.

People who can successfully recall dream content have been shown to display higher frequencies of EEG activity in their frontal areas, and less so in the parietal areas, when compared to people with no dream recall. This fact might be significant because, although dreaming requires low slow-wave activity in the posterior hot zone regions, remembering the dream may require involvement of the frontal parietal regions, which are also known to be important for working memory.

You're more likely to remember your dreams if you wake up briefly during or right after REM sleep. These awakenings help capture your dream's content.

Deciphering dreams

Modern dream interpretation really took off in the Victorian era when physicians began using dreams to understand psychiatric conditions like hysteria and other neuroses. Also, during this era, dream interpretation looked at how dreams might act to reveal unconscious desires, personality attributes, or conflicts, as well as how they might express underlying thoughts and fears.

Sigmund Freud, the pioneer

Sigmund Freud (the founder of psychoanalysis) was a neurologist who set up his clinical practice in Austria in 1886. As a pioneer in the field of dream interpretation, Freud linked dreams to ungratified instincts triggered during sleep. He proposed that these instincts, often related to unresolved desires, prompt the occurrence of dreams. He also suggested that many dreams take on a negative emotional tone rather than being neutral. He believed that apparently negative dreams disguise the direct gratification of sexual and aggressive instincts, which, if openly expressed, could disrupt sleep. To avoid this disruption, the dreamer's mind censors the dream by disguising the instinctual gratifications.

Freud believed that by examining a patient's dreams, he could uncover these wishes for gratification and understand how patients defensively managed them. He often asked his patients to engage in *free association*, a method by which they said whatever came to mind about their dreams. Even if the expressed associations seemed unrelated, Freud felt that they led back to the core impulses driving the dream.

REMEMBER

Freud often interpreted dreamers' instincts as being sexual in nature and used this lens for his analyses.

Carl Jung, the archetypist

Carl Jung, another influential figure in dream analysis, began practicing psychotherapy in Switzerland around 1907, initially collaborating with Freud. However, he had a different approach from Freud (see the preceding section). He believed that dreams reveal unconscious aspects of personality and conflicts, especially during adolescence.

Jung placed less emphasis on sexuality than did Freud, and he focused on archetypes, such as the mother figure. He believed that these archetypes influenced an individual's development and would manifest in dreams. Jung also introduced the concept of compensation, suggesting that if aspects of your personality, like thinking versus feeling, are unbalanced in waking life, they would appear in your dreams to restore balance.

REMEMBER

Unlike Freud, Jung preferred to interpret the content within the dream itself rather than rely on free association.

Alfred Adler, the wisdom seeker

Alfred Adler started practicing psychology in Austria in the early 1900s, and like Jung, initially collaborated with Freud. As another key dream analyst, he focused on inferiority complexes and how they drive behavior. He viewed dreams as a way to express underlying thoughts rather than disguise them. Adler believed that the struggles and fears you experience in dreams reflect those in waking life, and sometimes dreams provide insights that prepare you for future situations. He argued that by studying dreams, you could gain significant wisdom.

Modern approaches to dream analysis

In 1993, the International Association for the Study of Dreams published a statement on the ethics of dream work. They emphasized the importance of ethically studying dream images, feelings, and associations to help guide dreamers toward a deeper understanding of their dreams. Modern therapeutic approaches to dream interpretation often involve exploring how emotions, body sensations, or images in dreams relate to your waking life.

Today, dream interpretation continues to play a role in psychotherapy, with a focus on using systematic and supportive methods to enhance the therapeutic process. Research shows that patients often highly rate dream interpretation sessions, finding value in how these discussions strengthen the *therapeutic alliance* (the connection and collaboration between therapist and client) and lead to personal insights, even though not all earlier theories, such as those proposed by Freud, have received empirical support.

TIP

With a therapist, you may explore techniques such as replaying a dream with your eyes closed or inducing a trancelike state to help connect with the dream content more deeply.

Having Sensory Experiences in Dreams

Dreams often feel incredibly real because they mirror how your brain processes sensory information during waking life. Most dreams are primarily visual, and dreaming about familiar faces or scenes activates the brain areas responsible for sight perception when you're awake. Dreams can also involve other sensory experiences, including sound (auditory), touch (tactile), taste (gustatory), and bodily sensations (somatosensory). Additionally, *Wernicke's area*, a part of the brain that processes speech when you're awake, is also activated when you dream about conversations.

Dreaming and movement

You may dream of walking, running, or other physical activities, but your body stays still during REM sleep. Neurons in your brainstem suppress motor activity to prevent movement while you're sleeping. However, people afflicted with REM sleep behavior disorder (RBD) may act out their dreams, sometimes violently (see Chapter 8 for more about this disorder).

WARNING

Acting out your dreams can be a sign of REM sleep behavior disorder. If you notice this happening, consult a sleep medicine physician for help to ensure your safety while sleeping.

Awareness and consciousness in dreams

Most dreamers aren't aware that they're dreaming. You may feel like you're part of a story or scene but never realize that it's not real. This lack of awareness is likely due to decreased activity in the frontal-parietal regions of your brain, which normally help distinguish between sleep and wakefulness. However, if you experience *lucid dreams*, you can recognize that you're dreaming and even control parts of the dream. See the section "Knowing That You're Dreaming" later in the chapter for information about lucid dreams.

Emotions in dreams

Dreams often carry a heavy emotional tone. Brain scans show increased activation in the limbic and paralimbic areas — regions of the brain involved in processing emotions. You're more likely to remember dreams that have strong emotional content, especially those that make you feel intense emotions like fear, joy, or sadness.

TIP

If you wake up from a highly emotional dream, jot it down immediately. Keeping a dream journal can help you track recurring emotional themes in your dreams.

DREAM CONTENT AND AGE

Dream content significantly changes as you grow. as reported in research studies, kids aged three to five years old have fewer dreams when they wake up from REM sleep, and they report almost none from NREM sleep compared to older children and adults. These early REM dreams are usually brief and often lack complex social interactions, emotions, and self-descriptions, but they frequently feature animals and body-related themes.

As they grow older, children's dreams become more frequent and detailed. From ages five to nine, the length of dreams increases, and the content involves more interactions and body movements. In this age range, NREM dream reports also start to appear. By ages seven to nine, kids report even longer dreams in both REM and NREM sleep.

(continued)

(continued)

As a child's development continues, dreams evolve from simple, single scenes to more complex, time-linked sequences. By ages 9 to 11, REM dream reports become nearly as frequent as those of adults. Between ages 13 and 15, the largest increase in NREM dream reports happens. Existence of mental imagery and visual-spatial abilities — in contrast to language skills — correlate best with the frequency of dream reports.

Exploring Dreams and Mental Health Conditions

Dreams aren't just a fascinating psychological phenomenon; they can also provide valuable insight into your mental health. In psychology and psychiatry, understanding how dreams interact with anxiety, post-traumatic stress disorder (PTSD), depression, and other psychiatric disorders can help you manage your mental well-being more effectively. This section explores the connections between dreams and these conditions, offering insight into how your nighttime experiences can reflect and affect your mental health.

Disturbing dreams and anxiety disorders

Anxiety often involves anticipating danger or misfortune, accompanied by feelings of tension and discomfort. These symptoms become a clinical concern when they cross over into an anxiety disorder, which can significantly impair your quality of life. This category of disorders includes conditions such as

>> Phobias

>> Obsessive-compulsive disorder (OCD)

>> Panic disorder

>> Acute stress disorder

>> Generalized anxiety disorder

>> Anxiety disorders related to medical conditions or substance abuse

Studies have shown an association between anxiety and disturbing dreams, although findings can be mixed. Some research doesn't show a clear connection. One consistent finding is that individuals with anxiety disorders tend to experience

>> A reduction in the amount of time spent in REM sleep

>> An increase in the amount of time spent in NREM, stage N1 sleep

Because most dreaming occurs during REM sleep, the reduced time spent in that sleep stage might explain why the link between anxiety and disturbing dreams isn't always clear.

For those with OCD, some evidence suggests that dream content may reflect daytime symptoms and distress. Establishing a direct link between generalized anxiety and disturbed dreaming is challenging, because few studies have examined this connection specifically. However, effectively treating anxiety-related nightmares is crucial for improving both sleep quality and overall mental health.

Mimicking insomnia: PTSD

The psychiatric disorder *PTSD* typically involves exposure to a traumatic event that includes actual or threatened death, serious injury, or intense fear, helplessness, or horror. People with PTSD often

>> **Relive the traumatic event** via dreams, flashbacks, or even physical symptoms such as sweating or a racing heart

>> **Avoid trauma-related stimuli** that might trigger distressing memories

>> **Experience numbed responsiveness** and reduced ability to feel emotions

>> **Have heightened arousal,** causing feelings of being on edge and anxious

When it comes to sleep, PTSD often mimics insomnia, causing difficulty falling and staying asleep along with recurring distressing dreams of the traumatic event. Most people with PTSD experience these nightmares, which can also affect children, though the repetitive dream replay of the trauma might not be as obvious in kids.

Dreaming may be twofold with PTSD

Interestingly, you may experience both non-PTSD-related dreams following trauma and the more typical post-traumatic nightmares associated with PTSD. Some individuals report moving through traumatic images and emotions quickly before developing PTSD-associated dreams. Studies show that certain sleep-related phenomena — for example, recurring distressing dreams and sleep disturbances right after trauma — can lead to more severe, chronic PTSD symptoms later on.

REMEMBER

Nightmares in PTSD often result from heightened brain responsiveness to neu-rotransmitters like *norepinephrine*, a chemical messenger that increases at night. (See Chapter 4 for more information about neurotransmitters and sleep.) Indi-vidual vulnerabilities (mental illness, for example) can also contribute to the development of PTSD-related nightmares.

Several theories explain why PTSD-related dreams tend to be more severe:

>> Some experts believe these nightmares have an adaptive function, helping you gradually extinguish fear memories during waking hours by reliving them in your dreams.

>> People with PTSD often have greater *REM density* (a measurement of the number of eye movements during REM sleep) than do people who don't have the disorder. This increased REM pressure likely results from fragmented and shortened REM sleep, which disrupts emotional processing that normally may occur during REM sleep.

Investigating treatment for PTSD dreams

Image rehearsal therapy (IRT) is a common treatment for PTSD and other anxiety-related nightmares. IRT works by reducing the frequency and intensity of night-mares, which in turn decreases REM disruption. IRT involves

>> Rehearsing the nightmare content in a safe, controlled way

>> Creating catharsis through exposure to the disturbing dream content

>> Rewriting the storyline to reduce emotional impact

TIP

Exploring the underlying emotions, themes, and connections in your dreams can help integrate and connect traumatic events with existing memories, reduce dis-tress associated with the trauma and related negative emotions, and offer new insights that lessen the emotional burden of PTSD.

In cases where nightmares are a significant feature of mental health conditions like PTSD, medications such as prazosin and trazodone have been shown to be effective in helping to reduce the frequency of these disturbing dreams. Anxiety reduction strategies, including IRT, are effective, and even a single group session can provide relief.

REMEMBER

Addressing nightmares, especially those tied to traumatic experiences, can sig-nificantly improve your overall sleep quality and mental health. If your night-mares occur at a frequency of one or more per week, cause distress, interfere with your ability to fall asleep or stay asleep, impact your mood, or lead to daytime anxiety, talk to a sleep specialist about treatment options that could help reduce their frequency and intensity.

Depression and unpleasant dreams

Depression often involves *anhedonia* — a decreased interest in pleasurable activities. You may also experience symptoms (some of which are seemingly contradictory) such as

» **Weight changes,** either gaining or losing weight

» **Disrupted sleep** or an increase in the time you spend sleeping

» **Physical agitation** that results in increased physical activity, restlessness, and repetitive movements

» **Fatigue** that may be associated with irritability, lack of concentration, and reduced productivity

» **Feelings of worthlessness or hopelessness** and related negative views of yourself, the world in general, and the future

» **Thoughts of death or *suicidal ideation,*** a preoccupation with the idea of suicide

» **Difficulty concentrating** and other cognitive dysfunction such as slowing of the ability to learn and process information

Depressive disorders include major depressive disorder, dysthymic disorder, and depressive disorder not otherwise specified. Doctors make these diagnoses when symptoms reach a clinically significant level and cause distress or impairment of your daily functioning and quality of life.

How dreams relate to depression

Researchers have studied dreams and depression since the early 1960s, and study results show that unpleasant dreams occur more frequently in those experiencing depression when compared to those who don't. These unpleasant dreams often involve painful experiences, and even after depression resolves, many people continue to have the same types of unpleasant dreams. Studies have found that dreams in depressed individuals frequently include themes such as

» Deprivation, disappointment, or rejection

» Exploitation, mistreatment, or ridicule

» Punishment, physical injury, or feeling lost

If you're experiencing persistent disturbing dreams, especially those involving themes of death, suicide, or abuse, talk to a healthcare provider. These dreams can reflect your emotional state and are probably important to discuss in the context of your mental health.

Traits of depression-related dreams

Research consistently shows that people with depression report fewer and shorter dreams, with poor recall, especially if they're receiving medication for their depression. Dreams often feature fewer characters and display flattened emotions. Among those with severe symptoms of depression, dream content tends to be more restricted, and they may feel like an external observer rather than an active participant.

Depression-related dreams also have a reduction in visual sensory experiences, which contributes to this overall flattened dream content. Interestingly, some studies have found that if you report more negative dream content near the end of your sleep period, you might have a higher chance of remission from depression when you are reassessed a year later. This suggests that your dreams may play a role in processing and down-regulating depressed mood over time.

Other psychiatric disorders

Dreams are a significant focus in psychoanalysis and psychotherapy (areas associated with the early dream researchers are covered in the section "Deciphering dreams" earlier in the chapter), although dreams are less commonly used outside these settings. But dreams can still come into play when related to other mental disorders.

Psychosis

If you're experiencing *psychosis* (a mental disorder that causes you to lose touch with reality, characterized by symptoms such as hallucinations, delusions, and disorganized thinking and speech), you might also have mental experiences during the transition between wakefulness and sleep — known as *hypnagogia*.

The hypnagogia transition can include

>> **Sleep paralysis,** which makes you temporarily unable to move or speak

>> **Hallucinations,** which cause you to perceive something that's not really there

>> **Out-of-body experiences,** which give you the sensation of being outside your own body and observing yourself from a distance

These characteristics of hypnagogia can be mistaken for psychotic episodes in individuals without psychosis, especially when sleep paralysis includes hallucinations, such as feeling an intruder in the room or experiencing chest pressure or suffocation. Although these experiences can be frightening, they are often a normal part of sleep physiology and usually reflect REM sleep intruding into wakefulness — a time when vivid dreams and muscle paralysis naturally occur.

REMEMBER

If you have frequent sleep paralysis or vivid hallucinations that disrupt your sleep, discussing these experiences with a sleep medicine physician might help you find ways to manage them better.

ADHD

If you or your child has *attention-deficit/hyperactivity disorder* (ADHD), you or your child may have dream-related symptoms as well as the behavioral symptoms of inattention, hyperactivity, and impulsiveness. You might notice that dreams often involve negative themes such as threats, aggression, or misfortunes. These themes could be linked to the stress of managing ADHD or underlying biological processes.

Anorexia

Dreams in individuals who have *anorexia* (an eating disorder, typically with excessive weight loss that results in people weighing less than is considered healthy for their age and height) often feature cognitive distortions about body image and eating. These distortions reflect daytime struggles with these issues of perception.

RBD and parasomnias

REM *sleep behavior disorder* (RBD) causes people to act out their dreams, sometimes violently. This disorder often appears before conditions like Lewy body dementia or Parkinson's disease, and at least 10 percent of people with RBD also experience psychiatric symptoms. The dreams of people who have RBD frequently feature more aggressive content when compared to the dreams of those who don't have the disorder. See Chapter 8 for more information about RBD.

TIP

If you suspect you or a loved one has RBD — especially if there's sleep-related accidental violence — seeking a medical evaluation is crucial, because it can be linked to other health conditions.

Parasomnias, which are unusual behaviors during sleep, include sleepwalking, sleep terrors, nightmares, and sleep paralysis (see Chapter 8 to learn more about these disorders). If you or someone close to you experiences frequent parasomnias, especially following trauma such as physical or sexual abuse, they may be at increased risk of uncovering underlying psychiatric issues.

EMERGING THERAPIES

When managing psychiatric disorders, treatment often includes psychotherapy, behavioral therapy, and pharmacological approaches. Some newer therapies have unique effects on sleep and dreaming due to their impact on brain neurotransmitters.

Recently explored for treating conditions like depression and PTSD, psychedelics (like psilocybin) induce altered states of perception that mimic dreamlike psychotic episodes. These substances work through serotonin receptor activation in the brain, offering unique antidepressant and anti-anxiety effects that traditional therapies may not provide. Psychedelic therapy uses these altered states as part of treatment, showing promise for conditions that have been difficult to treat with conventional methods.

Known primarily as an anesthetic, ketamine has become a rapid-acting treatment for major depression, particularly when other antidepressants have failed. Unlike traditional medications that can take weeks to work, ketamine can reduce symptoms quickly and even acutely decrease suicidal thoughts. However, its effects aren't limited to mood — ketamine can induce visual and auditory hallucinations, trigger out-of-body experiences, and significantly alter sleep patterns by increasing total sleep time and affecting REM sleep.

These novel treatments like psychedelics or ketamine have the potential to significantly alter your sleep and dream experiences. Always consult with your healthcare provider to understand how these treatments might impact you.

In older adults, parasomnias may indicate or be mistaken for more serious conditions, such as seizures, brain tumors, or neurodegenerative diseases, so discussing these symptoms with a healthcare provider is important.

How Your Medication Influences Your Dreams

Various medications can influence the vividness, frequency, and nature of your dreams. Some drugs enhance the dream experience, while others suppress it or alter its content:

>> **Medications used to treat Alzheimer's disease,** as well as those specifically aimed at increasing dream vividness and lucid dreaming, can make your dreams more intense and memorable. Similarly, medications that provide

more dopamine to the brain treat conditions like Parkinson's disease and REM sleep behavior disorder and they may enhance the vividness of your dreams.

>> **Antidepressants, however, tend to have a variable effect.** Selective serotonin reuptake inhibitors (SSRIs) may suppress REM sleep due to increased serotonin levels, leading to sleep disturbances, vivid dreams, or nightmares.

>> **Beta blockers, often prescribed for hypertension, may induce vivid dreams or nightmares.** If you notice changes in your dream patterns while on these medications, discuss them with your doctor.

WARNING

Medications can significantly impact your dream experiences (either by altering the content or eliminating dreams altogether), but don't stop them without consulting a healthcare provider. Discontinuing medications that suppress REM sleep, such as antidepressants, can lead to a phenomenon called *REM sleep rebound*, where vivid dreams and nightmares become more frequent. This can also happen with substances like alcohol, where withdrawal can cause vivid hallucinations due to REM sleep intrusion. If you've recently stopped a medication and are experiencing disturbing dreams, speak with your healthcare provider for support and guidance on managing these symptoms.

Knowing That You're Dreaming

Lucid dreaming happens when you realize that you're dreaming while still asleep. After you become aware of the dream, you may be able to control the dream, which opens up opportunities for enhancing problem-solving, creativity, and even practicing skills for waking life. However, lucid dreaming occurs infrequently in most people and research studies evaluating lucid dreaming are limited.

How lucid dreaming works

Lucid dreams typically occur during REM sleep, particularly in its most active phases. During these lucid dreams, your heart rate, breathing, and rapid eye movements increase compared to other phases of REM sleep. Research to evaluate lucid dreams includes

>> **Movement pattern and dream matching:** Researchers can verify lucid dreaming by observing specific eye movement signals during sleep studies, such as the left-right-left-right-center (L-R-L-R-C) pattern. These eye movement patterns are prearranged between the researcher and the lucid dreaming individual prior to a sleep study. This arrangement allows scientists to match your reported dream content with the data recorded while you were asleep.

>> **Image processing insights:** Eye movement studies provide further insight into how your brain processes visual imagery during dreams. By signaling lucidity and then tracking objects within your dreams, such as tracing circles or following lines, your recorded eye movements may closely match the direction of your gaze in the dream. This suggests that what you see in a dream feels more like real perception than mere imagination.

Neuroimaging techniques such as functional magnetic resonance imaging (fMRI) reveal that during lucid dreaming, areas of your brain, such as the frontal-parietal brain regions, show increased activity similar to wakefulness. These areas usually quiet down during regular REM sleep, highlighting perhaps a distinct conscious state of lucid dreaming. Researchers have also explored how your dream actions might mirror waking movements. For example, when you clench your hands in a lucid dream, your brain's motor areas activate (though in a slightly weaker way) just as they would if you were awake.

Scientists also examined how people control their breathing in lucid dreams by having study participants in their dreams simulate tasks like diving underwater and for comparison, they also performed the tasks during waking imagination. These scenarios showed that you retain some cortical control over the irregular respiration during REM sleep, blending conscious control with the automatic processes of REM sleep.

Using lucid dreaming as a tool

Lucid dreaming can be more than just an interesting phenomenon — it can be a useful tool, especially if you're struggling with nightmares. When you realize you're dreaming, you might be able to change the nightmare's storyline, reducing its emotional impact. This approach, called *lucid dreaming therapy*, may be beneficial for those who experience frequent nightmares or PTSD.

If you have narcolepsy, you might notice that you experience lucid dreams more often. These dreams can provide psychological relief as you navigate your typically vivid and complex dream landscapes. Researchers are continually exploring methods to make lucid dreaming more accessible, because most people rarely experience lucid dreaming naturally.

Lucid dreaming may be a skill that can be learned. If you'd like to develop your lucid dream abilities, you might try

>> **Sleep interruption (wake-back-to-bed):** Wake up briefly during the night and then go back to sleep. Lucid dreams are more likely to occur after you return to sleep, especially during later REM cycles.

>> **Prospective memory techniques:** Set an intention to remember that you're dreaming by recalling past dreams and mentally practicing how to recognize dreamlike elements.

>> **External sensory cues:** Use sounds, scents, or tactile sensations to trigger awareness within your dream, helping you to recognize that you are lucid dreaming.

>> **Certain medications:** Galantamine, for example, which is used to treat Alzheimer's disease, has shown promise in research studies by increasing lucid dream frequency when combined with sleep interruption and memory techniques.

TIP

Start working toward lucid dreaming by keeping a dream journal and reviewing it regularly. Doing so helps you spot recurring themes and recognize when you're dreaming.

3

Dealing with Your Sleep Situation

Find out how to build better sleep habits and improve your sleep through diet, exercise, and routines for all life stages.

Explore common struggles such as difficulty falling asleep or feeling out-of-sync with your sleep schedule, and how to address them.

Uncover the characteristics of restless movements during sleep, unusual nighttime behaviors, breathing issues, excessive daytime sleepiness, and their treatments.

See how sleep medicine specialists diagnose issues and what to expect from a visit to a sleep center.

Chapter **6**

Getting Healthy Sleep

Getting healthy sleep isn't just about how much time you spend in bed — it's about paying attention to your body, your lifestyle, and the many factors that affect your sleep. By making small changes to your daily habits — from diet and exercise to screen time and stress management — you can improve the quality of your sleep and feel more alert, rested, and energized throughout the day.

I know you've probably heard this said before: "Just get eight hours of sleep, and you'll be fine!" Well, if only it were that simple, right? The truth is that your body is a bit more complex than this simple sleep-fix implies. You might be lying in bed for eight hours, but if your mind is racing or your room feels like a sauna, you most likely aren't getting the rest you need. Healthy sleep involves more than just hours logged in bed — the quality of those hours matters just as much as the quantity.

In this chapter, I not only help you figure out how to improve your sleep, but I also give you a clear idea of what's considered normal or typical when it comes to sleep patterns. After all, how can you recognize healthy sleep if you're not sure what it comprises? I take you through discovering how much sleep you really need to knowing what those restless nights might be telling you. And I help you explore how your diet, exercise habits, and even that late-night Netflix binge may be sabotaging your best sleep efforts. So grab your favorite cozy blanket (but maybe not too much caffeine) and delve into how to fine-tune your sleep routine for the best results.

Identifying Normal Human Sleep

Sleep is essential for human health, but what does *normal* sleep look like? Although sleep patterns vary from person to person, general guidelines and a basic structural organization — a *sleep architecture* — applies to most people.

A typical night's sleep follows a repeating cycle that lasts roughly 60–90 minutes (sometimes as long as 120 minutes) and moves through various stages of non-REM (NREM) and REM sleep. A sleeping person experiences

>> **NREM sleep,** which consists of stages N1 through N3, starting with light sleep (stage N1), progressing to slightly deeper sleep (stage N2), and ending with deep sleep (stage N3), also called *slow-wave sleep* or *delta sleep* (since it is comprised primarily of delta, or 0.5-4 Hz frequencies).

>> **REM sleep,** the stage in which most dreaming occurs, may play an important role in memory consolidation and emotional health.

If you have healthy sleep architecture, you cycle through these stages multiple times during the night, with the amount of deep sleep (N3) being higher earlier in the night and REM sleep increasing in the latter part of your night's sleep.

REMEMBER

But the sleep cycle doesn't always follow such a simple pattern because individuals can pass through sleep stages in a seemingly random order throughout the night. For example, some people can pass through the sleep stages in an order more like N1, N2, N1, REM, N2, and then N3. To read more about the states and stages of sleep, turn to Chapter 2.

Disruptions to sleep architecture — whether from stress, external noise, sleep or medical disorders, or lifestyle factors — can lead to fragmented sleep, which causes you to feel less refreshed even if you've spent sufficient time in bed.

Examining Sleep Differences

Women generally sleep longer than men. This difference in the amount of sleep starts early in life and persists through adulthood. Also, beginning in adolescence, women's circadian rhythms tend to shift (earlier in life than men's) to an *eveningness chronotype* (a preference for doing more tasks and activities in the evening and having a later bedtime). This shift causes women to be more prone to having both later bedtimes and wake-up times. Women also tend to report poorer sleep quality — which includes more difficulty falling and staying asleep — when compared to men.

Differences in sleep architecture by sex

Men and women have significant differences in sleep architecture according to sleep studies (polysomnography, see Chapter 9), which use brain wave activity (that doctors measure through EEG):

>> **EEG characteristics:** Differences in EEG activity become particularly noticeable during adolescence. In general, women tend to exhibit higher power in the distribution of electrical activity in NREM and REM across wide frequency bands, indicating higher neural activity in these sleep states. Researchers believe that this occurrence relates to anatomical differences, particularly in the *thalamus*, the part of the brain that processes a majority of sensory information and also plays a major role in sleep, wakefulness, and memory.

Women also have differences in their *sleep spindles* (waveforms 12–14 Hz that are most common in N2 sleep) versus those of men. These differences may give women an edge when it comes to the continuity of sleep and perhaps consolidation of memory.

>> **Slow-wave sleep:** Both girls and boys experience a drop in the amount of slow-wave sleep (N3 sleep) as they age, but the decline happens faster for boys, potentially due to differences in the timing of puberty.

- Girls tend to preserve slow-wave sleep for a longer period. In general, women often experience longer periods of slow-wave sleep than men, and researchers believe that these slow-wave periods are crucial for physical restoration. The advantage (of more slow-wave sleep) tends to diminish with age, particularly after menopause.

- Boys, on the other hand, experience a greater amount of light sleep, which increases the likelihood of frequent awakenings and fragmented sleep.

Hormonal changes affecting sleep

Once girls hit puberty, their hormonal changes, especially those related to the reproductive life cycle, can drastically affect their sleep:

>> **Premenstrual period:** Many women experience sleep disruptions in the days leading up to menstruation. Premenstrual periods often bring insomnia, due to fluctuations in estrogen and progesterone. These hormonal changes can result in restless sleep, and this pattern may worsen as women age.

>> **Pregnancy:** Sleep disturbances are common during pregnancy, particularly in the first and third trimesters. Hormonal shifts and physical discomforts — such as frequent urination, stress, back pain, leg cramps, and acid reflux — can significantly disrupt sleep. As you would expect, sleep studies during

pregnancy (particularly in the third trimester) tend to show lower amounts of total sleep, more awakenings, lighter sleep, and less deep and REM sleep in pregnant compared to non-pregnant women.

Many pregnant women develop restless legs syndrome (RLS) and obstructive sleep apnea (OSA), which further worsens their sleep quality. Also, increased risk for gestational diabetes and hypertension, preeclampsia, eclampsia, and low infant birthweight are sometimes associated with OSA during pregnancy.

TIP

Try managing pregnancy-related sleep disturbances by using pillows for extra support, practicing good sleep hygiene (see Chapter 15), and talking to a doctor about potential treatments for conditions such as insomnia, OSA, and RLS.

>> **Postpartum:** After giving birth, sleep fragmentation becomes a major problem for new mothers (to read more on sleep fragmentation, turn to Chapter 3) because it leads to stress and daytime dysfunction. Most mothers experience frequent awakenings due to the demands of caring for their infant, such as night feedings and diaper changes. This interrupted sleep can last up to eight months postpartum.

In addition to the external factors that disturb sleep, postpartum hormonal fluctuations can also disrupt sleep and contribute to postpartum depression (PPD). In particular

- *PPD has a bi-directional relationship with sleep,* meaning that poor sleep makes depression worse, and in turn, depression makes sleep more difficult and of lower quality.

- *Mothers with PPD often report more frequent awakenings and difficulty falling back asleep* after being woken by their baby. Evidence also suggests that infants born to mothers with PPD tend to have more disrupted sleep.

WARNING

PPD and related sleep problems can be life-threatening! If you're experiencing postpartum sleep challenges, talk to your doctor and seek support. Addressing sleep problems can significantly improve both your mental and physical health during the postpartum period.

>> **Menopause:** Women going through menopause often report a decline in sleep quality, mainly due to drops in the hormones estrogen and progesterone. These hormonal changes can lead to lighter sleep and a reduction in deep sleep, causing frequent awakenings throughout the night.

Women are also at a higher risk of developing insomnia during menopause, which may persist even after menopausal symptoms subside. Hot flashes and night sweats — hallmarks of menopause — can further contribute to sleep disturbances. These sudden episodes of intense heat can wake women multiple times during the night, leading to sleep fragmentation and daytime fatigue.

TIP If menopause is affecting your sleep, talk to a healthcare provider about strategies to manage hot flashes and hormonal fluctuations, such as hormone replacement therapy (HRT) or alternative treatments.

Sleep disorder differences by sex

Differences in sleep for the different sexes are also evident when it comes to sleep disorders. Table 6-1 lists common sleep disorders and their comparative prevalence by sex. To read more about the symptoms, diagnosis, and treatment of all sleep disorders regardless of sex, turn to Chapters 7 and 8.

TABLE 6-1 **Sleep Disorder Prevalence**

Sleep Disorder	Higher Prevalence In	Facts
Insomnia	Women	Women are at higher risk for insomnia than men (especially during periods of hormonal changes when it is known as *menstrual-related insomnia, pregnancy-related insomnia*, and *menopausal insomnia*); depression or anxiety disorders (which are more frequent in women) may also lead to poor sleep quality
Nightmares and hallucinations	Women	Women report experiencing nightmares and hallucinations more frequently (especially during adolescence and young adulthood), perhaps due to having better dream recall than men, higher rates of anxiety and depression, and sex-specific socialization (learning sex roles, attitudes, and behaviors expected in a specific culture starting at birth and throughout life)
Obstructive sleep apnea (OSA)	Men	More common in men than women, but OSA increases in women after menopause to be almost as frequent as in men, which is likely due to a protective effect of progesterone and estrogen on the maintenance of muscle tone of the upper airway (lost at menopause); compared to men with OSA, women tend to experience less OSA severity (but more REM-related sleep-disordered breathing) and are more likely to have mood disturbances and hypothyroidism (that can worsen their OSA symptoms)
REM sleep behavior disorder	Men	Higher in prevalence in men (especially among those over 50 years of age, when it is the most common); may be more common in men due to hormonal differences; it is associated with neurodegenerative diseases like Parkinson's disease (which is more common in men)
Restless legs syndrome (RLS)	Women	Twice as common as in men, but risk significantly increases in women during pregnancy and worsens with subsequent pregnancies; compared to men with RLS, women have more difficulty falling asleep and periodic limb movement disorder (PLMD) more commonly occurs

REMEMBER

If you believe that you're experiencing any sleep disorders, discussing your symptoms with a healthcare provider is important. Women and men may present differently when it comes to conditions such as sleep apnea or insomnia, so don't hesitate to seek proper diagnosis and treatment.

Racial and ethnic sleep differences

Sleep quality and duration don't just vary from person to person or by sex — they also differ across racial and ethnic groups. Research suggests that racial minorities, in particular, are more likely to experience sleep disruptions and shorter sleep durations. That finding might come as a surprise, but understanding differences based on race and ethnicity is the first step toward addressing them:

>> **Black, Native Hawaiian/Pacific Islander, and multiracial/multiethnic individuals** tend to report the highest prevalence of less than seven hours of sleep per night. Of these groups, Black-identifying individuals appear to sleep less per night compared to white-identifying individuals, as confirmed by both subjective, self-reported data (like a questionnaire) and objective data (gathered through polysomnography and actigraphy, for example).

>> **Latinx/Hispanic and Asian populations,** particularly individuals of Chinese descent, also report shorter sleep durations.

>> **Black and Mexican American individuals** are also more likely to report greater than nine hours of sleep than white individuals.

>> **East Asians** have more severe OSA than that of their white counterparts when they have similar body mass indices, indicating that their upper airways may be more collapsible due to differences in craniofacial structure.

>> **Black, Hispanic, and Mexican American populations** demonstrate a significantly higher risk of OSA when compared to white populations. For instance, Black children are four to six times more likely to develop OSA when compared to white children. In addition, the prevalence of severe OSA symptoms is higher in these groups.

>> **Black and Native American/Native Alaskan individuals** report poorer sleep consistent with insomnia compared to white individuals. Hispanic populations report higher rates of RLS than white populations, while Chinese Americans show lower rates of RLS. These differences might have roots in both genetics and environmental factors.

Even though providers recommend treatments (and they're available), cultural differences can influence how effectively people use them. For example, CPAP *nonadherence* (the refusal or inability to stick with CPAP therapy for OSA) is more common among Black individuals compared to their white counterparts. Research points to several related factors, including communication from healthcare providers, the patient's understanding of the treatment, and personal attitudes toward CPAP therapy.

Cultural practices around sleep also play a significant role in shaping behaviors:

» **Co-sleeping and bed-sharing:** According to a 1984 research study, about 70 percent of Black versus 35 percent of white families report sharing a bed with their infants. In contrast, in a 2002 study, the incidence of parent-child co-sleeping in Korea was 88 percent. (See the sidebar "What about co-sleeping?" also in this chapter for more about this.)

» **Napping:** In many Mediterranean and Latin American countries, midday naps are customary. For example, as reported in a 2000 study, 72 percent of adults in Brazil report taking at least one nap per week, compared to 55 percent of adults in the U.S. (National Sleep Foundation 2005 Sleep in America poll.)

TIP

Cultural and ethnic differences can influence your sleep habits and behaviors. Always seek personalized solutions for your sleep issues — especially if you feel your healthcare provider isn't fully addressing your concerns.

Knowing Whether You Get Enough Sleep

As I mention in the chapter's introductory paragraphs, getting enough sleep isn't just about the number of hours in bed. Quality, consistency, and how you feel during the day are all critical factors that define whether your sleep is adequate. Doctors generally recommend that adults aim for about seven to nine hours of sleep each night, but individual people's needs vary based on factors such as age, lifestyle, and overall health.

How much sleep do you really need?

Your sleep requirement is as personal as your fingerprint. Some people naturally function well with less than seven hours of sleep, and others may need closer to nine hours. The goal is to figure out what amount of sleep works best for you. Just because your partner or friend thrives on less sleep doesn't mean that your body will do the same.

To make attaining your sleep goal a bit more interesting, the amount of sleep you need also changes as you age. Here are some typical age-related sleep ranges:

>> **Newborns:** 14–17 hours per day

>> **Children:** 9–12 hours per night

>> **Adolescents:** 8–10 hours per night

>> **Adults:** 7–9 hours per night

>> **Elderly:** 7–8 hours per night

But what happens if the amount of sleep you get regularly falls outside of these typical ranges? The distinction between short sleep and long sleep becomes important in this discussion. While sleep patterns can vary, consistently getting too little or too much sleep may be a red flag signaling possible sleep disorders or other health issues.

To break down the distinction

>> **Short sleep (six hours or less):** Research shows that consistently sleeping less than six hours per night increases your risk of serious health conditions, such as coronary heart disease, stroke, obesity, diabetes, mental health issues, and even *all-cause mortality* (the total number of deaths from any cause). This relationship between short sleep and serious health conditions can go both ways. Short sleep can contribute to the onset of these health problems, but existing medical conditions — such as chronic pain or anxiety — can also lead to shorter sleep.

>> **Long sleep (nine hours or more):** Regularly sleeping more than nine hours is also linked to poor health outcomes, including diabetes, hypertension and other cardiovascular conditions, obesity, and cognitive decline. People who report long sleep durations often experience underlying health conditions such as depression or sleep apnea, which can extend the overall time they spend asleep.

REMEMBER

Both short and long sleep often connect to underlying issues, rather than being causes for atypical sleep duration by themselves. If you find that you regularly sleep less than six hours or more than nine hours and feel tired, checking in with a healthcare provider to find out whether an underlying medical condition could be affecting your sleep is worthwhile.

Clues that you're not getting enough sleep

If you're waking up tired despite getting enough hours of sleep, you should evaluate your sleep environment, nighttime habits, and overall sleep quality. Are you waking up refreshed, or do you feel groggy and tired throughout the day? Some people may function well on the lower end of the typical range of sleep hours, while others need more sleep to feel their best. Even though feeling tired is a pretty common occurrence, don't shrug it off, especially if the feeling is persistent.

WARNING

Chronic sleep deprivation can lead to serious long-term effects, including a higher risk for heart disease, diabetes, and depression.

The best way to know if you're getting enough sleep is by paying careful attention to how you feel during the day after a night's sleep. Here are some clues:

>> **Cognitive impairment:** Poor attention, memory issues, or difficulty concentrating may be signs that you need more sleep. Lack of sleep affects vigilance, learning, and higher-order cognitive functions, such as driving a car or making complex decisions at work.

>> **Daytime sleepiness:** You shouldn't feel excessively sleepy during the day if you're getting enough sleep. Falling asleep during meetings, while driving, or while reading can be a major sign of sleep deprivation.

>> **Near accidents or microsleeps:** If you've experienced near misses or accidents due to momentary lapses into sleep (*microsleep* is the technical term for the situation in which your brain shifts from wake to sleep for a few seconds), this could be a strong sign that you need to improve your sleep duration or quality.

WARNING

If you experience a microsleep and close your eyes while driving — even for a few seconds — the result could be a fatal accident. Officers typically use information from accident scenes to determine the causes of accidents. For example, finding no skid marks shows that the driver wasn't applying the brakes, and the conclusion might be that they likely experienced a lapse of consciousness — like a microsleep.

>> **Mood changes:** If you notice that you're more irritable, moody, depressed, or anxious, you may not be getting sufficient sleep.

>> **Physical signs:** Sudden weight gain or increased hunger could indicate that your sleep quality is poor. Sleep affects your appetite-regulating hormones (such as ghrelin and leptin), and your appetite may increase. Turn to Chapter 3 to read more about how those hormones work.

TIP

If you experience any of the sleep-deprivation clues noted in this section, try increasing your sleep by 15-minute increments each week. For example, if you currently sleep 7 hours but still feel sleepy, try going to bed 15 minutes earlier and maintaining your usual wake time for a week. Continue this process (of increasing sleep time by 15 minutes for a week, while maintaining wakeup time as the anchor) until you no longer feel sleepy during the day. If adding segments to your sleep time doesn't work to improve daytime sleepiness, you may need to consider that your issue isn't the quantity of sleep, but the quality of sleep instead.

Managing the Balance Between Nutrition, Exercise, and Sleep

Your body's overall health intricately connects to how well you sleep. And nutrition and exercise directly affect your sleep quality. When you understand how each of these elements interacts with your sleep, you can make better choices to optimize your rest.

The impact of diet on sleep

What you eat doesn't just fuel your day — it also plays a key role in how well you sleep at night. Although large-scale research studies are lacking in this area, certain foods may help you drift off faster, while others may leave you tossing and turning.

Improving your overall diet

You can follow these suggestions for an overall diet improvement:

>> **Eat foods rich in unsaturated fats,** such as olive oil, nuts, and seeds, to promote deeper, more restorative sleep.

>> **Eat high-fiber foods,** such as beans, broccoli, berries, and avocado to reduce nighttime awakenings and increase deep sleep.

>> **Try the Mediterranean diet,** because it features fruits, vegetables, legumes, fish, and healthy fats, and helps to boost both sleep quality and duration.

>> **Avoid or limit saturated fats,** such as dairy products and red meat because they often lead to lighter sleep and daytime fatigue.

>> **Avoid refined sugars and processed foods,** which can cause fluctuations in blood sugar levels and affect your energy and alertness throughout the day.

>> **Try to avoid large meals, especially those high in simple carbohydrates, close to bedtime.** Ironically, many people often feel sleepy after a big meal full of carbs (this is called *postprandial sleepiness*), so it would seem to make sense to do it right before bed, but that's a no-no for quality sleep. Specifically,

- *Foods with a high glycemic index* (meaning they raise blood sugar quickly) can shorten the time it takes you to fall asleep, but they often come with a catch — lower-quality sleep.

- *Large, heavy meals late at night* may lead to indigestion and gastroesophageal reflux, which can make falling asleep harder to do.

Stick with lighter, balanced dinners at least two to three hours before bedtime — otherwise, you may find yourself waking up more frequently and getting less deep sleep overall (especially after an epic dinner, like you have on Thanksgiving or other holidays).

Eating foods that may help you sleep

TIP

Speaking of Thanksgiving (see the previous bullet list), you've probably heard that *tryptophan* — an amino acid — helps you sleep by boosting serotonin and melatonin levels. But here's the twist: Turkey isn't actually the best source! Foods such as cheddar cheese, pumpkin seeds, and even chocolate (though it also contains caffeine!) pack more of a tryptophan punch than does turkey. Plus, eating high-carbohydrate meals can make tryptophan more effective by helping it cross the blood–brain barrier.

Some research shows that a few other foods enhance sleep quality by reducing *sleep latency* (the amount of time needed to fall asleep) or increasing overall restfulness:

>> **Tart cherry juice:** Some studies show that tart cherry juice (which is packed with melatonin) may improve sleep duration and sleep quality.

>> **Kiwi fruit:** High in serotonin and melatonin, kiwi may help you fall asleep faster and improve sleep efficiency.

>> **Fatty fish:** Thanks to its rich content of omega-3 fatty acids and tryptophan, fatty fish such as sockeye salmon may help improve your sleep quality.

TIP

Everyone responds differently to foods, so try experimenting with sleep-friendly snacks. For example, eat a small handful of nuts or a banana with almond butter before bed; keep trying to see what works best for you.

REMEMBER

The effects of vitamins, minerals, herbs, plant extracts, and other dietary supplements for improving sleep have not been examined in-depth nor in many research studies. Supplements that may improve sleep include vitamin D, magnesium, and valerian. However, data to support the use of these supplements are limited, and because these over-the-counter (OTC) products are not approved by the U.S. Food and Drug Administration you should be cautious and consult with your physician before taking them.

Children and nutrition

What your child eats can have a big impact on their sleep. Kids who regularly eat a balanced breakfast (that includes protein, whole grains, healthy fats, and fruits, for example) tend to enjoy better sleep quality and show a preference for morning routines. On the flip side, skipping breakfast or eating erratically is linked to delayed sleep onset and poorer overall sleep quality.

For infants, breastfeeding plays an important role in how quickly they consolidate their sleep patterns. Breast milk changes composition throughout the day, with nighttime feedings being higher in carbohydrates and tryptophan — both of which promote sleepiness. These elements help establish and regulate the infant's circadian rhythm more effectively than formula-fed infants and encourage longer, more restful sleep at night.

REMEMBER

Establish regular mealtimes for your children, especially in the morning. Starting the day with a nutritious breakfast can set the tone for healthier sleep patterns and better overall rest.

Shift workers and nutrition

If you're a *shift worker* (an employee whose work schedule falls outside the standard hours of roughly 9 a.m. to 5 p.m.), maintaining a healthy sleep-wake cycle can be tough. The irregular hours often lead to circadian rhythm misalignment, which can make falling asleep and waking up at consistent times harder to do. However, your diet can help — careful meal planning can support your body's alertness during shifts and promote sleep afterward.

TIP

Avoid heavy meals during night shifts, because they can make you feel sluggish and interfere with sleep later. Instead, opt for light, balanced snacks that keep you energized without overloading your system. Eating consistent, well-balanced meals or snacks at the same time each day can help align your circadian rhythm and improve your overall sleep quality — whether you're working during the day or at night.

Obstructive sleep apnea and diet

OSA is a condition that causes interrupted breathing during sleep. It's closely tied to weight and overall nutrition. If you're dealing with OSA, managing your weight through a balanced diet and regular exercise can improve both your overall health and sleep quality.

Individuals with OSA tend to have higher levels of the appetite-stimulating hormone ghrelin and the hunger-regulating hormone leptin. They may

>> **Often develop leptin resistance,** which contributes to overeating and weight gain.

>> **Commonly report weight loss after they start CPAP** (continuous positive airway pressure) therapy. But studies show mixed results regarding whether CPAP alone leads to weight loss.

>> **Respond to medications containing glucagon-like peptide-1 (GLP-1),** a hormone that helps regulate blood sugar and appetite. For example, tirzepatide (Zepbound), a GLP-1 medication, is FDA-approved to treat adults with moderate-to-severe OSA and obesity.

Alcohol, caffeine, and cannabis

The nonfood substances we consume — whether alcohol, caffeine, or cannabis — can have profound effects on the quantity and quality of our sleep. In this section, you find out how each one of these substances interacts with your sleep cycle.

Assessing alcohol

Alcohol may help you fall asleep quickly, but it negatively impacts your sleep quality as the night goes on. Research shows that alcohol's effects on sleep are similar for both men and women. However, women may be more vulnerable to alcohol-related sleep issues due to differences in how their bodies process it.

Alcohol has these effects on sleep:

>> **At first, it acts as a sedative** by enhancing *GABA inhibition* (a neurotransmitter effect; see Chapter 4 for more information) and reducing *glutamatergic excitation* (that is, the neurotransmitter glutamate decreases the normal stimulating action of the nerve cells in the brain). These effects help you fall asleep faster, especially at low doses.

>> **It can lead to sleep problems during the second half of the night.** In general, while alcohol can increase slow-wave sleep (N3) during the first few hours, it also leads to sleep fragmentation and REM sleep disturbances later on, making you wake up more frequently.

WARNING

If you have insomnia, you might be tempted to use alcohol as a sleep aid. However, over time, you can develop a tolerance to its sedative effects. This means that while alcohol might help at first, it eventually becomes less effective, and long-term use can actually lead to chronic sleep problems.

Carefully consuming caffeine

Caffeine is great for getting through the day, but it can wreak havoc on your sleep if you're not careful with how much and when you consume it. Caffeine blocks *adenosine receptors*, which are responsible for making you feel sleepy as the day goes on. By blocking these receptors, caffeine reduces *sleep pressure* (the daily build-up of the urge to sleep), meaning that caffeine can result in you taking more time to fall asleep. It also decreases slow-wave sleep, which is essential for physical recovery.

Caffeine can temporarily improve your cognitive performance (primarily by its effects that boost alertness) and help you fight daytime sleepiness — especially after a night of bad sleep. However, if you're well-rested, caffeine may not have much of a positive effect on your cognitive performance.

WARNING

Please heed these warnings regarding the intake of caffeine:

>> **Having caffeine too late in the day can seriously interfere with your sleep.** Consuming caffeine within 6 hours of bedtime can reduce your total sleep time and increase *sleep latency* (the time it takes to fall asleep). Research shows that having caffeine from 30 to 60 minutes before bedtime cuts down on deep sleep (N3) and leads to more awakenings after sleep onset.

>> **Drinking more than three cups of coffee (or other caffeinated beverage) per day can lead to chronic sleep disruptions,** shorter sleep times, and daytime sleepiness. Regular caffeine use can also mask underlying sleep problems (such as daytime drowsiness due to obstructive sleep apnea) that need to be addressed.

TIP

Limit your caffeine intake to two or three cups of a caffeinated beverage per day, and avoid drinking the beverage after early afternoon (say, 2:00 p.m.) to prevent it from interfering with your sleep. The *half-life* (the length of time required for half of a substance to be eliminated from the body) of caffeine is approximately 5 hours.

Considering cannabis (CBD and THC)

Cannabidiol (CBD) exists along with delta-nine-tetrahydrocannabinol (THC) in the cannabis sativa plant. Both of these compounds are psychoactive (they affect the mind), but CBD comes without the potential for substance abuse. Many people commonly use CBD for pain, depression, anxiety, and as a sleep aid, but the scientific evidence to definitively support its effectiveness for treating sleep problems and disorders is lacking.

Research on how CBD affects sleep is still in its early stages, and currently, not enough proof exists for me to recommend it as a go-to treatment for insomnia. Some early studies show that CBD may help reduce sleep disturbances at a dosage around 160 mg, but more placebo-controlled trials are needed to confirm its benefits. In addition, studies looking at THC in combination with CBD reveal that the combination reduces slow-wave sleep at low doses but increases wakefulness at higher doses.

REMEMBER

Always consult your healthcare provider before using CBD or THC to help with sleep. Their effects vary between individuals, and long-term research on their impact is still limited.

How exercise affects sleep

Exercise is one of the most effective ways to improve sleep quality. Researchers don't fully understand the mechanism by which exercise helps sleep, but they suspect that it may work by shifting the timing of the sleep-wake cycle in a favorable direction or improving depression or anxiety symptoms that may hinder sleep. Both acute (short-term) and chronic (long-term) exercise can positively impact your sleep, by reducing insomnia-like symptoms, decreasing sleep disruptions, and increasing total sleep time. However, different types of exercise, as well as the timing and intensity, play a role in the specific benefits you experience.

Trying out acute exercise

A single bout of moderate-intensity exercise can have immediate effects on your sleep, but timing and duration matter.

Acute exercise improves total sleep time, time to REM sleep, and amounts of N2 and slow-wave sleep (N3) — the deep sleep stage crucial for physical restoration. However, the time of day when you exercise makes a difference. For example, exercising

>> **Within four hours of bedtime** may delay sleep onset and cause sleep fragmentation.

>> **Within four to eight hours before bedtime** reduces sleep latency and decreases waking periods during sleep.

>> **For more than one hour** tends to have a stronger impact on the total sleep time, although this extent of exercise may not be practical for everyone.

REMEMBER

High-intensity exercise right before bed may disrupt sleep, particularly if you're new to exercising; however, some data indicates that exercise may improve sleep latency and depth.

Choosing chronic exercise

In the long run, regular (chronic) exercise leads to significant improvements in sleep, especially for older adults and those struggling with sleep disorders like ongoing insomnia. After about four months of regular exercise, individuals report better overall sleep quality. Consistently exercising over time may improve

>> **Sleep onset:** You may be able to fall asleep more quickly

>> **Total sleep time:** Giving you a longer sleep duration

>> **Daytime alertness:** Boosting your attention throughout the day

TIP

Target your exercise to your sleep needs. Certain types of exercises — such as yoga, tai chi, and relaxation-based exercises — are particularly effective for improving sleep quality, especially with older adults. These activities tend to be more beneficial for promoting restful sleep than are higher-intensity workouts such as aerobics or resistance training.

Sleep disorders and the role of exercise

For individuals with sleep disorders such as insomnia, OSA, and RLS, practicing consistent, moderate-intensity exercise is key to improving both symptoms and sleep quality. Specifically, you may find that

>> **Regular moderate-intensity exercise has been shown to reduce insomnia symptoms.** Exercising in the late afternoon tends to provide the best results, improving total sleep time and sleep efficiency, and reducing sleep latency.

>> **Regular exercise can help reduce the severity of OSA by at least 25 percent, even without significant weight loss.** Exercise may strengthen the muscles in the upper airway, which helps prevent airway collapse during sleep — a common issue in OSA.

>> **Moderate-intensity exercise also helps reduce the severity of RLS and periodic limb movements during sleep (PLMS).** However, exercising too close to bedtime may worsen sleep quality, as well as RLS symptoms in some people, so it's best to exercise earlier in the day.

Optimizing Sleep for Your Age Group

Sleep needs change as people age, and what works for one age group may not be as effective for another. Tailoring sleep habits to different life stages ensures that you get the most restful, restorative sleep possible for all stages. In this section, you can find out how to optimize sleep for children, adolescents, adults, and the elderly.

For a child

Children's sleep patterns change dramatically as they grow. Infants initially sleep in *polyphasic patterns*, meaning they sleep in short periods throughout the day and night. Over time, their sleep consolidates into longer stretches at night.

The following are some specifics about sleep characteristics for children:

>> **Newborns sleep around 14 to 17 hours per day,** but their sleep is fragmented. As they grow, a child's sleep consolidates into longer nighttime sleep, eventually becoming *monophasic* (one main sleep period) in early childhood.

WARNING

You should place infants on their backs at bedtime, with the face and head clear of blankets or other soft items to reduce the risk of sudden infant death syndrome (SIDS).

>> **Naps are crucial for young children,** not just for physical rest, but for cognitive development. Regular naps improve memory retention and emotional regulation. Skipping naps can lead to irritability, decreased alertness, and poorer performance on cognitive tasks.

>> **Children's sleep needs change as they age.** At ages 2–5 years, they need about 11–13 hours of sleep per night, while school-aged children (ages 6–12 years) need 9–12 hours.

>> **Children thrive on routine.** A predictable bedtime ritual helps signal that it's time to wind down. A good routine may include a warm bath, story time, or light breathing exercises. However, no right answer exists for children who have difficulty adapting to a sleep routine and adhering to a regular bedtime schedule.

WHAT ABOUT CO-SLEEPING?

Co-sleeping is a very common practice in which family members sleep together, whether sharing a sleeping surface (bed) and/or sleeping in the same room. This practice occurs more commonly in certain countries (such as those in Asia). No long-term positive or negative psychologic effects for the practice of co-sleeping as a lifestyle choice seem to exist.

For *reactive co-sleeping* (in which the parent is present as a response to child's sleep difficulty), limited data exist, but co-sleeping with children aged two to four years may predict a lower risk of bad dreams when they reach five to six years old. Breastfeeding and co-sleeping are common, and breastfeeding studies have indicated that infants who are breastfed have a significantly lower risk of SIDS.

However, given the potential risk of co-sleeping and SIDS, the American Academy of Pediatrics Task Force on Sudden Infant Death Syndrome and the Committee on Fetus and Newborn recommends that infants sleep in the parents' room, close to the parents' bed, but on a separate surface designed for infants, ideally for at least the first six months.

One popular method for encouraging children to find a path to sleep comes from pediatric sleep expert Dr. Richard Ferber. The method he developed is called *graduated extinction sleep training*, which involves letting your child cry for short periods and then returning to the child's bedroom at specific check-in intervals. These intervals gradually lengthen each night, with the goal of having the child develop self-soothing skills that enable them to independently fall and stay asleep.

WARNING

Parents should prioritize keeping an eye on their infant's and children's sleep, because those who obtain insufficient sleep or have sleep disturbances may experience a variety of issues. These include delayed cognitive development; problems with attention; emotional concerns, conduct- and peer-related problems; and increased body weight. They may also develop psychiatric problems such as depression, anxiety, or ADHD (or be at risk for this diagnosis). ADHD specialists may not systematically ask about sleep. If sleep improves, a dramatic decrease in ADHD symptoms often occurs. So before any final ADHD diagnosis or start of treatment, specialists should include questions about sleep in the evaluation process.

For an adolescent

Adolescents (age 13 to 18) sleep an average of 8–10 hours per night. However, due to busy school and family schedules, many adolescents get fewer hours of sleep.

During adolescence, the body's internal clock shifts in a way that makes falling asleep early and waking up in time for school more difficult. This natural circadian phase delay can result in chronic sleep deprivation for this age group.

Here are some other notable facts about sleep for adolescents:

WARNING

» **Because adolescents tend to stay up later and prefer to sleep in, this sleep-wake schedule can conflict with early school start times.** The circadian shift that they experience is due to natural hormonal changes and delayed melatonin release, which can lead to sleep deprivation during the week. Fortunately, a nationwide movement is underway to delay school start times with the goal of improving sleep and (consequently) daytime alertness, especially in adolescents.

Keep an eye out for signs of sleep deprivation (such as excessive daytime sleepiness). Chronic sleep deprivation is linked to higher risks of depression, anxiety, and poor academic performance. Sleep loss also affects emotional regulation and decision-making.

» **Adolescents often try to make up for lost sleep by sleeping in on weekends.** However, oversleeping on weekends can disrupt their circadian rhythms and make maintaining a regular sleep schedule harder to do. Similarly, napping can also offset the sleep-wake schedule and negatively affect the ability to fall asleep at bedtime.

» **Adolescents may try to compensate for lost sleep in other ways.** Using substances such as caffeine and alcohol (which they shouldn't have at all) can make adolescents' sleep quality and quantity worse. Cutting off consumption of these substances a few hours before bedtime minimizes their deleterious effects on sleep.

TIP

Blue light from screens can interfere with melatonin production, which can delay sleep onset and reduce overall sleep quality. Encourage your adolescents to set a screen-time curfew and avoid using smartphones, laptops, TVs, and other electronic devices for at least an hour before bed to ensure proper melatonin production. Also encourage them to keep consistent sleep and wake times, even on weekends, to regulate their body clock and improve sleep quality.

For an adult

Adults often struggle to balance sleep with work, family, and social responsibilities. Many fall short of the recommended seven to nine hours of sleep, which can lead to chronic sleep debt. (See Chapter 3 for more about sleep debt.) Adults cycle through NREM and REM sleep throughout the night. However, factors such as stress, poor diet, and lifestyle choices (such as alcohol or caffeine consumption at inappropriate times) can often disrupt sleep. And chronic stress can lead to insomnia, in which individuals struggle to fall asleep, or wake frequently during the night. Cortisol, the stress hormone, stays elevated and prevents relaxation.

TIP

Prioritize stress management techniques such as meditation, deep breathing, or yoga to improve sleep. Reduce alcohol and caffeine intake, especially in the evening. Also maintain a consistent sleep schedule, create a relaxing bedtime routine, and ensure that your sleep environment is comfortable.

Outlining sleep changes for adults

When you examine sleep throughout adulthood, you find that total sleep time progressively declines. You also find a corresponding increase in wakefulness after sleep onset, which results in lower *sleep efficiency* (proportion of time someone is asleep while they're in bed).

Here are some specifics related to the sleep experience in adults:

>> **Adult sleep is lighter:** They experience a decrease in deep slow-wave (N3) sleep, an increase in lighter stages of sleep (N1 and N2), and REM sleep tends to hover at around 25 percent of total sleep time from the mid-20s on. As adults age, their circadian sleep-wake system gradually becomes less robust with poorer quality of sleep at night and more drowsiness during the day. Adults also have a decreased ability to rebound from nights of either partial or total sleep loss compared to when they were younger.

>> **Sleep (and other) disorders become more prevalent and disruptive to sleep:** Disorders such as OSA, RLS, and chronic insomnia occur more frequently in adults. (See Chapters 7 and 8 for more complete coverage of sleep disorders.)

Other medical disorders can also arise and take the form of hypertension, heart disease, thyroid disease, chronic obstructive pulmonary disease (COPD), gastroesophageal reflux disease (GERD), chronic pain, type 2 diabetes, and cancer. Also, mental conditions such as depression and anxiety can disrupt sleep during adulthood.

For women, menopause may lead to poor sleep and development of OSA (independent of body mass index). Additionally, hot flashes, night sweats, and depression that can accompany menopause in adult women may further worsen sleep by leading to frequent awakenings and insomnia. Medications such as hormone replacement therapy, and selective serotonin reuptake inhibitors (SSRIs) can improve sleep during menopause.

>> **Many medications prescribed for adults to treat any of these sleep, medical, or psychiatric disorders may potentially worsen sleep:** For example, stimulants prescribed for the daytime sleepiness of narcolepsy, bronchodilator medications for asthma, and some antidepressants can negatively affect sleep.

Dos and don'ts for healthy adult sleep

Check out Table 6-2 for some important dos and don'ts for healthy sleep as an adult.

TABLE 6-2   **Sleep-Related Dos and Don'ts for Adults**

What to Do	How to Do It
Do	
Maintain a healthy lifestyle	A healthy diet and regular exercise regimen promote sleep and stable circadian sleep-wake rhythms.
Establish a regular sleep-wake schedule	Go to bed near the same time each night and awaken near the same time each day for all days of the week. Keeping wakeup time constant is especially critical.
Allow adequate sleep time	Make time for at least 7 hours of sleep per night.
Set up a conducive sleep space	Make sure that your bedroom matches your preferences for temperature, noise level, mattress and pillow firmness, and light exposure.
Use light to synchronize your body's sleep-wake cycle	Within 5 minutes of awakening, go outside (into the sunlight) or stay in an indoor area that receives significant sunlight for 30 minutes to align your sleep-wake cycle with your desired awakening time. If you typically awaken before dawn, applying a UV-filtered light box (10,000 lux and 18" from eyes) is an acceptable substitute for sunlight. Conversely, avoid bright light for a few hours before bedtime to prevent it from delaying your sleep onset.
Establish a regular relaxing pattern before sleep	Meditation, yoga, or a warm bath can help to promote sleep.
Create and manage a *worry list*	A few hours before bedtime, write down all the items that are bothering you to serve as a *placeholder* for the worries. (You don't have to deal with them immediately, but don't forget to address them.) This practice can lessen the chance that these worries flood your mind the moment your head hits the pillow.

(continued)

TABLE 6-2 *(continued)*

What to Do Don't	How to Do It
Engage with stimulating substances and activities close to bedtime	Avoid exercise, caffeine, nicotine, alcohol, heavy meals, or heavy liquid intake for at least two hours before bedtime.
Take OTC medications that you haven't vetted	Discuss any OTC medication with your healthcare provider. Note: An exception would be melatonin; a 0.3 mg dose of melatonin may help those who have symptoms of insomnia.
Watch TV or read in bed	Avoid these activities unless they definitely make you drowsy.
Work in bed	Avoid activities that require mental effort or may cause stress — like working. Also, avoid using a smartphone, tablet, or computer (even with blue-blocking software) at least 30 minutes before bedtime.
Nap during the day	Power through the day without naps so that you avoid affecting your night's sleep. You may take a short nap (10 to 20 minutes) to avoid driving when drowsy, and taking a nap at the same time of day for a set amount of time is okay because your body will become used to taking this daily nap. Enhance the benefits of this short nap by taking caffeine just prior to the nap, which allows the caffeine to enter your system and help with alertness.
Linger in bed longer than 20 minutes if you can't fall asleep (or back to sleep)	Get up and go to another room, do something that makes you drowsy (meditation, for example), and then go back to bed when you feel drowsy. This is important for reconditioning your body to associate the bedroom as a place to sleep.

For the elderly

The good news for older adults is that the decline in total sleep time (as well as N3 and REM sleep) and the ability to fall and stay asleep appears to plateau at about the age of 60 years. The bad news is that wakefulness after sleep onset increases and the ability to fall asleep continues to decrease with advanced age.

Older adults typically need around seven to eight hours of sleep, although as people age, sleep efficiency declines, and older adults experience more fragmented sleep. Older adults often feel sleepy earlier in the evening and wake up earlier in the morning; this *advanced sleep phase* represents a normal shift in the timing of their circadian sleep-wake rhythm.

WARNING

Although older adults appear to be more resilient to the effects of sleep loss than younger adults, older adults who regularly sleep less than six hours have increased risk of cognitive dysfunction and mortality. Additionally, an association between excessive daytime sleepiness in the elderly and subsequent cognitive decline and dementia is suggested.

Dealing with more prevalent medical and psychiatric conditions

As people age, they're more likely to develop medical issues (musculoskeletal pain) and psychiatric conditions (anxiety or depression) that interfere with sleep quality and duration. And like younger adults, older adults often face sleep disorders such as OSA, RLS, and chronic insomnia, which make getting restorative sleep harder to do. Managing these conditions with medication can also affect your sleep. Here are some aspects that relate to using medications to treat the conditions that older people might develop:

>> **Discuss with your doctor about using the lowest possible dose** of medication that still works effectively but minimizes side effects.

>> **Ask about medications that are more sedating (rather than alerting)** if you need to take them near bedtime

>> **Avoid medications that increase nighttime bathroom visits** so that they are less likely to cause frequent urination at night.

>> **Review the half-life of any medication** that could cause daytime drowsiness with your doctor.

Adopting the sleep recommendations for younger adults

To optimize your sleep if you're an older adult, you can look to the recommendations for younger adults. Specifically, older adults should

>> **Maintain a consistent sleep schedule** even though retirement may eliminate the pressure to go to bed and wake up at specific times — no alarm clock needed!

>> **Address sleep-disrupting conditions like OSA** to minimize fragmentation of sleep.

>> **Practice relaxation techniques** to reduce night-time wakefulness.

>> **Possibly introduce short, strategic naps (those that last no longer than 30 minutes),** which can improve alertness and mood without disrupting nighttime sleep.

WARNING

Long or frequent naps may worsen insomnia, and can disturb your normal sleep-wake rhythm.

Be sure to get your mental health regularly assessed, especially if you have lost some of your social support system due to death of loved ones. Compared to younger adults, maintaining regular physical activity and exercise (for example, walking or stretching), and light exposure during the day, are even more important for older adults because of the alterations in sleep and circadian rhythms that accompany normal aging. Regular physical and social activity can improve sleep quantity and quality in older adults, including those who are residing in nursing homes.

Chapter **7**

Sleeping Not Enough, Too Much, or Out of Rhythm

t's 2 a.m., and you're restless again. No matter how you toss and turn, comfort eludes you. You're exhausted, yet sleep seems impossible. Why is this happening? And more importantly, is there any way to get the relief you desperately seek?

This chapter offers clear, accessible explanations of sleep conditions, from how to identify symptoms to understanding the causes of various conditions such as insomnia, narcolepsy, and circadian rhythm disorders. When you understand, you can seek appropriate treatment.

If you're reading this in search of relief from your own (or a loved one's) sleep challenges, you're not alone. In this chapter, I offer medical insight, yes, but also hope that you can get the rest you need and live your fullest life. Sleep is not only a biological necessity, but also a gateway to vitality and health.

If you or a loved one has just received a diagnosis of a sleep disorder, you can use this chapter as a gentle guide to understand more about the condition and how to navigate the path of care.

Fighting Sleep: What Is Insomnia?

People of all ages can suffer from *insomnia*, which is the inability to fall and/or stay asleep. Insomnia is one of the most common sleep disorders. According to the Centers for Disease Control and Prevention (CDC), about one-sixth of all Americans may suffer from it. For people with insomnia, the condition often has a significant impact on their daily life, mood, and overall health.

TIP

Insomnia can be chronic (persisting over time), or acute (occurring briefly and then going away, often due to specific stressors).

You can find many associations and risk factors for insomnia:

>> **Poor sleep habits:** Those with insomnia can often have sleep habits that aren't conducive to sleep, such as failing to go to bed at roughly the same time every night.

>> **Medical conditions** (for example, heart or lung disease, or pain syndromes): These conditions can make falling asleep difficult and/or cause awakenings during the night.

>> **Life stressors:** These include divorce, loss of a loved one, changing jobs, moving to a new residence, and so on.

>> **Circadian rhythm sleep-wake disorders:** These disorders can be associated with insomnia; for example, delayed sleep phase disorder can make individuals have difficulty falling asleep at their usual bedtime.

>> **Medications:** For example, corticosteroids and certain antidepressants, such as fluoxetine (Prozac) or venlafaxine (Effexor) can cause sleep disturbances.

>> **Other sleep disorders:** For example, restless legs syndrome (RLS) and obstructive sleep apnea (OSA) — both of which you find out about in Chapter 8 — can result in difficulty falling asleep and staying asleep, respectively.

>> **Psychiatric disorders:** For example, anxiety, depression, and other disorders can be associated with insomnia; the disorders can cause insomnia, and insomnia can a worsen the disorders.

CAN YOU DIE FROM INSOMNIA?

The short answer is no. Fatal familial insomnia is an extremely rare, *neurodegenerative* disorder, which involves specific areas of the brain. Specialists have identified genetic mutations responsible for the disorder, and they believe less than 100 families in the world carry this mutation.

So the good news is that you are unlikely to have this mutation. The bad news is that the disorder is always fatal, typically within six years. It initially presents with symptoms of difficulty falling and staying asleep with episodes of falling into sleep and then acting out dreams, which progresses to coma and eventually death.

Recognizing symptoms of insomnia

The symptoms of insomnia disorder — whether chronic or acute — include

>> **Difficulty falling or staying sleep:** You are unable to fall asleep within 30 minutes after you turn off your bedroom lights or you have awakenings during the night and are unable to easily fall back asleep.

>> **Waking up earlier than you desire:** Your alarm is set for 7:00 a.m., but you can't sleep past 5:30.

>> **Resisting appropriate sleep-wake schedule:** You have difficulty going to bed on a sleep-wake schedule that is relatively consistent across days and nights, and is appropriate for your work and family activities.

>> **Requiring another party's involvement:** Kids (and others who are dependent) have difficulty sleeping without parent or caregiver interaction.

Getting diagnosed with insomnia

When you visit your doctor or a sleep specialist (check out Chapter 9 for ideas about interacting with a sleep specialist) because you think you might have insomnia, they take a patient history to understand your sleep habits and symptoms, and they may look at any sleep logs (or diaries) you have kept (see Chapter 9 also for information on sleep logs).

Doctors also perform a physical exam on your body to look for any anatomical reasons behind your sleeplessness — for example, large tonsils that might obstruct your airway — or other signs that suggest other sleep conditions (such as a peripheral neuropathy, which can be associated with restless legs syndrome) that can lead to poor sleep. They may also draw blood to check for several things, such as your thyroid condition and electrolyte levels. If either of those readings are abnormal, this may indicate a condition that can negatively impact your sleep.

REMEMBER

Typically, doctors don't perform in-lab sleep studies on patients with insomnia symptoms (unless they suspect other coexisting sleep disorders) because the sleep study reveals just what you'd expect: that the patients have difficulty falling asleep or maintaining sleep, and the sleep is mainly light rather than deep sleep.

The American Academy of Sleep Medicine established diagnostic criteria in their International Classification of Sleep Disorders that specialists use to diagnose chronic insomnia disorder. These include the following observations:

>> You or someone else observes that you experience at least one of the symptoms of insomnia (see the earlier section "Recognizing symptoms of insomnia").

>> You or your bed partner (or a caregiver) observes one or more of the following related to nighttime sleep difficulty: fatigue or malaise; impaired attention, concentration, or memory; impaired behavior in social, family, occupational, or academic activities; mood disturbance or irritability; daytime sleepiness; behavioral problems such as impulsivity (for example, gambling), aggression, or hyperactivity; reduced motivation and decreased energy or initiative; proneness to errors or accidents; and concern about or dissatisfaction with sleep.

>> Your symptoms aren't due to *inadequate opportunity*, which means that you don't allow enough time for sleep. When sleep specialists diagnose insomnia, they always assume that the patient allows at least seven hours for sleep if they're a healthy adult. Also, your sleep environment should be safe, dark, quiet, and comfortable for sleep. If it's not, your sleeplessness may be due to *inadequate opportunity*. For example, if you sleep in a very noisy environment or have a restless bed partner who disturbs your sleep, you are not providing an adequate opportunity for sleep.

>> You experience sleep disturbance and associated daytime symptoms (see those listed in a previous bullet point regarding nighttime sleep difficulty) at least three times per week. This sleep-wake difficulty and daytime symptoms must occur at this frequency (three times per week), be present for at least three months, and not result solely from another current disorder or medication/substance use.

REMEMBER

If you experience sleep disturbance and associated symptoms for less than three months, you aren't suffering from chronic insomnia disorder. But you may be suffering from an acute or short-term insomnia disorder. The diagnostic criteria for short-term insomnia disorder are identical to those of chronic insomnia disorder except for the duration of the symptoms, namely less than or three months or more, respectively.

Other diagnoses exist in which individuals don't meet the full diagnostic criteria for either chronic or short-term insomnia disorder. For example, excessive time in bed is an isolated symptom in which the individual takes a while to fall asleep — or has extended wakefulness periods during the night — but doesn't complain of insomnia or have daytime issues, such as fatigue or sleepiness. Lastly, a normal condition is a short sleeper, an individual who sleeps less than six hours per night, doesn't voluntarily restrict sleep but simply requires less sleep, has no issues of sleep difficulties, nor has any daytime issues.

HOW ACUTE INSOMNIA CAN BECOME CHRONIC

Sometimes, acute insomnia can lead to chronic insomnia when a person who has been a fairly good sleeper for most of their life experiences a traumatic mental, emotional, or physical event. An example could be something like going through a divorce or getting fired from a job. Due to the distress, the person starts experiencing poor sleep. If they don't receive prompt treatment for their poor sleep a behavioral pattern can set in, even after the original event resolves.

Doctors think that a traumatic behavioral event might somehow affect the neurons and neurotransmitters in the brain, and that's what may push acute insomnia into becoming chronic. But they don't fully understand why or how this occurs. Doctors consider this phenomenon to fit into the concept of psychophysiological insomnia — or biobehavioral insomnia — in which psychological or behavioral events can subsequently result in abnormal neurophysiologic or biologic processes.

Another example of an acute insomnia that can become chronic are those that sometimes appear following an infectious disease such as Lyme disease or COVID-19. Additionally, an individual may have an insomnia that seems to have been with them from day one without explanation. When doctors talk to these individuals, they frequently say, "Well, I haven't had a good night's sleep for decades." And for those patients, it is not unreasonable to think that a very early physiologic change may have somehow affected their sleep.

Receiving treatment for insomnia

Doctors use two primary types of treatment for insomnia. Specifically, they focus on behavioral therapy and prescribe medication. The next two sections outline these treatments.

Looking toward behavioral therapy

The main (and really, only) long-lasting treatment for chronic insomnia is *cognitive behavioral therapy for insomnia* (CBT-I), which involves several techniques that you can see in Table 7-1. Keep in mind, though, that no catch-all treatment exists. Your sleep specialist works with you to determine which specific mix of techniques is right for you, and they track your progress over time. Doctors use CBT-I regularly to treat insomnia because it's not only effective in the short term, but also has long-term, lasting effects.

TABLE 7-1   Cognitive Behavioral Therapy for Insomnia (CBT-I)

Technique	Goal
Circadian therapy	Synchronizing sleep-wake patterns to natural biologic rhythm
Cognitive therapy	Focusing on minimizing thoughts and beliefs that interfere with sleep
Relaxation training	Decreasing physical and mental stress/anxiety regarding sleep and awakenings from sleep
Sleep hygiene	Encouraging good sleep habits
Sleep restriction	Enhancing consolidation of sleep by reducing time in bed
Stimulus control	Reassociating the bedroom environment as the stimulus to ideal sleep

TIP

When you discuss treatment for insomnia with your doctor, work closely with them and keep an open mind. If you've been suffering from chronic insomnia for a while, you may be tempted to try to rule out ideas on your own, but I caution you not to.

Resist the urge to look up CBT-I and other behavioral treatment techniques online and automatically rule them out before talking with your sleep specialist. The best way to evaluate whether a treatment is appropriate for you is to have a psychologist trained in behavioral sleep medicine or CBT-I to meet with you to conduct an initial evaluation. Then have regular visits to decide which of the different methods or protocols within CBT-I are best for you to try.

Opting for treatment with medication

Doctors do use some medications to treat acute insomnia because medications typically only provide short-term results. The medications are enough to break the insomnia cycle before it develops into chronic insomnia, but aren't effective long-term due to dependence and tolerance (for example, your body gets used to the medication, resulting in the need for higher doses — typically until you reach the dosing limit). You can see some medications that doctors typically use to treat acute, or short-term, insomnia in Table 7-2.

WARNING

Some insomnia medications have serious side effects that increase in intensity if a patient stays on the medication too long.

TABLE 7-2 Commonly Prescribed Medications for Acute Insomnia

Medication	Typical Dose (mg)	Time to Peak Plasma Concentration (hours)	Half-life (hours)
Zolpidem (Ambien)	5–10	1.6	2.6
Zolpidem CR (Ambien CR)	6.25–12.5	1.5	2.8
Zaleplon (Sonata)	5–20	1	1
Eszopiclone (Lunesta)	2–3	1	6
Ramelteon (Rozerem)	8	0.75	2–5
Suvorexant (Belsomra)	10–20	2	12
Lemborexant (Dayvigo)	5–10	1–3	17–19
Daridorexant (Quviviq)	25–50	1–2	6–10

REMEMBER

You should avoid over-the-counter (OTC) medications for insomnia (and also medications like some antihistamines that have sedative properties) until you discuss them with your doctor, since some of them have been shown to have unfavorable side effects (for example, confusion/decreased cognition in the elderly, or falling). An exception is melatonin, which has been shown to combat insomnia in some individuals, especially if they have a *concomitant* (naturally associated) circadian rhythm sleep-wake disorder (most commonly, delayed sleep wake disorder). See the section "Sleeping When Everyone Else Is Awake" later in the chapter for more on circadian rhythm disorders. *Note:* Keep in mind that the FDA doesn't regulate melatonin, so if you decide to use melatonin, ensure that you obtain it from companies that you trust or find to have a good reputation.

Some medications that specialists prescribe for insomnia have their main indication for something else — for example, a sedating antidepressant such as trazodone. You should discuss taking these medications in detail with your doctor, because they may not want to prescribe a sedating antidepressant for an individual who has insomnia but not depression.

WARNING

CBT-I is the most effective long-term treatment for insomnia as compared to medications, so the use of a medication should be short-term. Don't stay on insomnia (or any) medications longer than your doctor prescribes; sometimes the side effects are too unpleasant or risky to experience long-term. Even OTC options such as melatonin can stay in your system the next day and cause you to feel carryover effects. If you've been on medication for insomnia for a long time and stop using it, you will invariably experience a *rebound* insomnia (especially if you stop it abruptly), so make sure to discuss gradually tapering off the medication with your physician.

THE DIFFERENCE BETWEEN FATIGUE AND SLEEPINESS

On the surface, fatigue and sleepiness might seem like the same thing, but they aren't, and understanding the difference between the two is key to understanding insomnia.

Fatigue is tiredness and a lack of energy and motivation, while sleepiness is feeling like you are going to actually fall asleep and have *microsleeps* (that is, a short period of sleep, typically less than 15 seconds). People with insomnia typically fit into the fatigue category because while they feel rundown and tired, even if they have the opportunity to sleep (whether during the day or night), they can't. And typically, these are the individuals in the waiting room of the sleep clinic who, instead of being totally asleep (like many patients are), mill about and read all the pamphlets or magazines. This is because people with insomnia experience an almost hyperarousal state from their insomnia.

Patients with insomnia have prolonged sleep latency (the time between when the lights go off and the person falls asleep). Plus, they have frequent awakenings throughout the night, and they're unable to fall back asleep, which increases their *wake after sleep onset*, which is one of the measures that doctors look at in the sleep lab. Additionally, they have decreases in both NREM (non-REM) and REM sleep, with the tradeoff of increases in light sleep, and although this light sleep prevents them from feeling sleepy during the day, it isn't enough to prevent them feeling fatigued.

Feeling Sleepy All the Time: Hypersomnia

Sleep specialists use the American Academy of Sleep Medicine's International Classification of Sleep Disorders to divide *hypersomnia* (extreme daytime sleepiness despite getting what should be adequate amounts of sleep) into a variety of individual disorders.

Nodding off with narcolepsy

Narcolepsy is a rare chronic neurological disorder that disrupts the brain's ability to regulate sleep-wake cycles effectively, and according to the National Institute of Neurological Disorders (NINDS), it affects about 135,000 to 200,000 Americans. People with narcolepsy often experience a blurred boundary between sleeping and waking states, which makes it difficult for them to control when they sleep. Narcolepsy has two peaks of onset: One happens typically in the teenage years, and the other happens in middle age (45 to 64 years). Additionally, doctors divide narcolepsy into two main types logically named type 1 and type 2.

Recognizing symptoms of narcolepsy

The symptoms of narcolepsy that show up (and disrupt) people's lives include

>> **Overwhelming drowsiness** (also known as *hypersomnolence*), which leaves the person feeling sleepy most of the time.

>> **Sudden sleep attacks,** which are irresistible and uncontrollable periods of sleep where the person suddenly and abruptly falls asleep.

>> **Sudden muscle weakness** during periods of strong emotion such as laughter, anger, or surprise. This condition is known as *cataplexy*.

>> **Hallucinations,** which happen more commonly when the person falls asleep (hypnagogic) rather than when they awaken from sleep (hypnopompic). The hallucinations can be visual, auditory, or somatic (for example, feeling like they're levitating off the bed or someone is touching them).

>> **Sleep paralysis** in which the person is paralyzed for a few seconds or minutes, usually when awakening from sleep.

>> **Disrupted nocturnal sleep,** in which people People who experience this symptom usually report that their sleep is very fragmented or disturbed.

Getting a diagnosis of narcolepsy

When trying to diagnose your sleep condition, a sleep specialist (see Chapter 9 for information about finding a sleep specialist) conducts clinical evaluations and specialized testing to assess your sleep patterns and brain activity. These may include

>> **Polysomnogram (PSG):** An overnight sleep study that records various physiological functions during sleep, including brain waves, heart rate, breathing, muscle activity, oxygen content, and eye movements. This test helps to rule out other sleep disorders. (See Chapter 10 for more on how this test works.)

>> **Multiple sleep latency test (MSLT):** A test that takes place the day after the PSG to measure how quickly you fall asleep in a dark and quiet environment during the day and how quickly and often you enter REM sleep. (See Chapter 9 for more on the MSLT.)

>> **Orexin-A level measurement:** A test that measures the level of orexin-A (also known as hypocretin-1) in the cerebrospinal fluid (CSF) by lumbar puncture (spinal tap). Low levels of orexin-A are particularly indicative of type 1 narcolepsy.

>> **Epworth Sleepiness Scale:** A questionnaire that you fill out yourself to help measure your general level of daytime sleepiness, which helps your doctor determine the severity of your condition. (You can find out more about questionnaires in Chapter 9.)

TIP

These tests, combined with a detailed medical history and symptom assessment, help your doctor diagnose narcolepsy and distinguish it from other conditions that can cause excessive daytime sleepiness.

Your sleep specialist diagnoses you with type 1 narcolepsy if

You have daily symptoms of a strong need to sleep or daytime sleep periods for at least three months.

You also have cataplexy and excessive sleepiness on the MSLT with two or more *sleep-onset REM periods* (SOREMPs) on the MSLT or one SOREMP in the preceding night PSG), and/or

You have a low orexin-A level in your CSF.

Your sleep specialist diagnoses you with narcolepsy type 2 (also known as narcolepsy without cataplexy) if

You have the same daytime sleepiness symptoms and sleep study findings as narcolepsy type 1 except you don't have cataplexy, either an orexin-A level from your CSF has not been measured or is normal, and

Your symptoms and/or sleep study findings are not better explained by other causes.

Excessive sleeping with idiopathic hypersomnia

Idiopathic hypersomnia is a condition in which you experience an ongoing need for excessive amounts of sleep for no apparent reason. It's not a result of other health issues, other sleep disorders, or outside influences.

Recognizing symptoms of idiopathic hypersomnia

You might have idiopathic hypersomnia if you

>> **Sleep a lot** (10 hours or more) at night but still feel very sleepy during the day.

>> **Take long naps** (1 hour or more) that don't make you feel refreshed.

>> **Find it hard to wake up from sleep,** and you often feel groggy.

>> **Have difficulty functioning during the day** because of sleepiness.

>> **Don't have** *cataplexy* (sudden muscle weakness associated with strong emotions).

Getting diagnosed with idiopathic hypersomnia

To diagnose idiopathic hypersomnia, your doctor

>> Asks about your sleep habits and whether you have a family history of sleep disorders.

>> Reviews your sleep diary or log if you have one. (See Chapter 9 for information about keeping a sleep diary or log.)

>> Performs a 24-hour PSG (*polysomnogram*; see Chapter 10) or conducts *wrist actigraphy* (which uses a wearable wrist device that measures sleep and wakeful states by wrist movements over time) in association with a sleep log — kept for at least seven days of unrestricted sleep — that averages total sleep time for the covered timeframe.

>> Performs an MSLT (*multiple sleep latency test;* see Chapter 9).

For your sleep specialist to diagnose you with idiopathic hypersomnia, you must have

Daily periods of irrepressible need to sleep or lapses into sleep occurring for at least three months.

No cataplexy, PSG and MSLT findings not consistent with a diagnosis of narcolepsy type 1 or 2, and a mean sleep latency of eight minutes or less on the MSLT and/or a total 24-hour sleep time of 660 minutes or greater (typically 12-14 hours) on 24-hour PSG or by wrist actigraphy with a sleep log.

No evidence of Insufficient sleep syndrome resulting from confirmed inadequate time in bed to sleep, and the hypersomnolence and sleep study finding can't be better explained by another disorder or medication/substance use.

Facing the rare Kleine-Levin syndrome

Kleine-Levin syndrome is a rare disorder in which you have repetitive periods of extreme hypersomnolence (excessive daytime sleepiness) that occur with behavioral (or psychiatric) and cognitive disturbances. For example, your daytime sleepiness may be accompanied by periods of excessive eating.

Recognizing symptoms of Kleine-Levin syndrome

You might have Kleine-Levin syndrome if

>> You find yourself sleeping most of the day and night during episodes that last about 10 days.

>> During these periods, you have unusual behaviors such as eating a lot, craving sex, feeling depressed, and having hallucinations and delusions.

>> Between episodes, you feel normal, with usual sleep and daily behavior.

Getting a diagnosis of Kleine-Levin syndrome

For your specialist to diagnose you with idiopathic Kleine-Levin syndrome, you must have

At least two recurrent episodes of excessive sleepiness and sleep duration, each persisting for two days to five weeks

Episodes that usually recur more than once a year and at least once every 18 months

Normal or near normal sleep and wakefulness, cognition, behavior, and mood between episodes, at least during the first years of the syndrome

Cognitive dysfunction, *derealization* (feeling detached from your surroundings, which may seem distorted or unreal), major apathy, and/or disinhibited behavior (for example, hypersexuality or hyperphagia) during the episodes

Hypersomnolence and related symptoms that are not better explained by other disorders or medication/substance use

Evaluating other hypersomnia

Hypersomnias can also be due to medical disorders (for example, Parkinson's disease), psychiatric disorders (such as bipolar II disorder), or medication use (sedatives) or withdrawal (stimulants). Other conditions that manifest as needing too much sleep are insufficient sleep syndrome and long sleepers (described in the next two sections).

Insufficient sleep syndrome

A sleep specialist may diagnose a patient with insufficient sleep syndrome if

The patient experiences an irrepressible need to sleep or daily episodes of falling asleep at inappropriate times (if it occurs in children before puberty, these symptoms might present as complaints of being more tired or having behavioral issues).

Their total sleep time is less than what they typically expect for the patient's age (via history, sleep logs, or actigraphy).

The abnormal sleep pattern is present on most days for at least three months.

Patients use alarms or are awakened by others to restrict sleep.

Patients tend to sleep longer on weekends or vacations.

Symptoms resolve when total sleep time is extended or are not better explained by other disorders or medication/substance use.

Long sleepers

Long sleepers are individuals who naturally sleep more than the average person in their age group. For adults, that's typically 10 or more hours of sleep per 24-hour period. This trait is usually an isolated symptom or a normal variation, as long as the individual does not meet diagnostic criteria for other hypersomnias.

REMEMBER

A long sleeper doesn't voluntarily extend their sleep, but simply requires more sleep, and has no other sleep difficulties or daytime sleepiness issues.

Treating hypersomnias

For hypersomnias, lifestyle adjustments are a crucial part of treatment. You must establish a regular nighttime sleep schedule and stay mindful of substances such as alcohol and medications that could affect your sleep.

Scheduling behavioral naps is also an important way to counteract hypersomnias, and your doctor can provide school excuses for enabling adolescents to take naps during lunchtime (usually in the nurse's office). And for an adult, the doctor can provide work-related exceptions so that you can take naps in your office settings.

TIP

As much as possible, try to stick to a regular bedtime and awakening schedule, and foster consistent sleep habits, including avoiding spontaneous naps and smartphones too close to bedtime.

In addition to good, regular sleep, some medications can help treat hypersomnias. These include

>> **Modafinil (Provigil) and Armodafinil (Nuvigil):** Stimulants that primarily increase dopamine in the brain. They are FDA-approved for treating excessive daytime sleepiness in adults with narcolepsy.

>> **Sodium oxybate:** Treats excessive daytime sleepiness and cataplexy in children and adults. There are three main formulations of sodium oxybate: the regular preparation (Xyrem), a lower-sodium option (Xywav), and a once-nightly formulation (Lumryz).

Currently, you find only one FDA-approved treatment for idiopathic hypersomnia, which is the low-sodium formulation of sodium oxybate.

>> **Solriamfetol (Sunosi):** Medication that works by increasing dopamine and norepinephrine in the brain and is FDA-approved for treating excessive daytime sleepiness in adults with narcolepsy.

>> **Pitolisant (Wakix):** Medication that affects histamine in the brain and is FDA-approved for treating excessive daytime sleepiness and cataplexy in adults with narcolepsy.

>> **Amphetamines/Methylphenidate:** Stimulants that enhance the activity of the central nervous system, particularly affecting dopamine, norepinephrine, and serotonin levels. Amphetamines and methylphenidate (Ritalin) are commonly prescribed to treat excessive daytime sleepiness in narcolepsy for both adults and children.

All medications, including these, have side effects. You should discuss these medications and side effects in detail with your sleep specialist.

OTHER DISORDERS THAT MAY AFFECT YOUR SLEEP

Your sleep specialist will undoubtedly consider other sleep-related medical and neurological disorders when evaluating your sleep problems. These include, but are not limited to, sleep-related

- Epilepsy (recurrent seizures during sleep)

- Headaches (headaches, such as migraines, occurring during sleep or awakening from sleep)

- Laryngospasm (spasm of the vocal cords, which causes difficulty breathing and subsequent awakening from sleep)

- Gastroesophageal reflux (reflux of gastric contents typically causing awakenings from sleep)

- Myocardial ischemia (decreased blood flow to the heart muscle during sleep)

Sleeping When Everyone Else Is Awake: Circadian Rhythm Sleep-Wake Disorders

Circadian rhythm sleep-wake disorders occur when your internal body clock, which regulates your sleep-wake cycle, doesn't align with the external environment. This situation causes problems such as insomnia or excessive sleepiness at inappropriate times. You can experience these disorders when events — traveling or changing work hours, for example — disrupt your natural sleep-wake patterns.

Recognizing symptoms of circadian rhythm disorders

If you recognize symptoms of circadian rhythm sleep-wake disorders in yourself, bed partner, or child, you should seek help. Do not try to tough it out on your own or think it will just go away. If these symptoms persist, you may need treatment.

Delayed sleep-wake phase disorder

When you have delayed sleep-wake phase disorder, you struggle to fall asleep and wake up at your desired (or required) times, and this pattern persists for over three months. You notice that when you follow a schedule that suits your internal clock, your sleep improves. If you could sleep when you prefer to, all would be okay.

Advanced sleep-wake phase disorder

With advanced sleep-wake phase disorder, you feel sleepy early in the evening and wake up unusually early — a situation which may become problematic for your daily routine. In this disorder, the skewed sleep timing also persists for more than three months and disrupts your life. When you can adjust your schedule to go to sleep earlier and get up at a still-early time (in order to match your internal clock's schedule), your sleep improves.

But the timing may be causing problems in your life, such as missing social activities or work opportunities that occur later in the evening. For the elderly (who are most affected by advanced sleep-wake phase disorder) living with younger family members, the very early morning activity in the house can cause disruption in the family.

Irregular sleep-wake rhythm disorder

If you have irregular sleep-wake rhythm disorder, you experience a scattered pattern of sleep-wake times over a 24-hour period. This pattern is marked by prolonged periods of wakefulness at night and prolonged sleep periods during the day that interfere with your daily life and persist for more than three months. This scattered pattern of sleep often indicates an underlying issue with your brain's sleep regulation (for example, a brainstem lesion), so you should seek the advice of a sleep specialist — especially if you have a sudden onset of this abnormal sleep-wake pattern.

Non-24-hour sleep-wake rhythm disorder

The non-24-hour sleep-wake rhythm disorder gives you sleep-wake periods that shift later (or earlier) each day. You may be sleepy during the day when you want (or need) to be awake and be awake at night when you want (or need) to be asleep. You experience symptomatic periods followed by asymptomatic periods for at least three months. This alternating-periods situation is due to your body's circadian sleep-wake rhythm not aligning with the environmental 24-hour light-dark cycle.

Shift work disorder

If your schedule requires you to work during typical sleep periods, you might find that sleeping when you need to is difficult. This situation can lead to insomnia and/or excessive sleepiness, less total sleep time, and impaired wake-time functioning. If these symptoms are present for three months, you may want to seek help to develop coping strategies and countermeasures for managing the work schedule.

Jet lag disorder

Jet lag disorder can happen following air travel across at least two time zones. You face insomnia or excessive daytime sleepiness, less total sleep time, and impaired daytime functioning. These symptoms emerge soon after your flight (that is, within a day or two).

Figure 7-1 depicts the sleep periods associated with some of the circadian rhythm phase shift disorders.

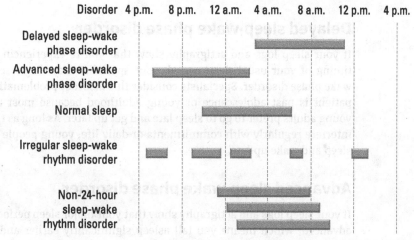

Sleep Periods for Circadian Rhythm Sleep-Wake Disorders

Disorder: 4 p.m. 8 p.m. 12 a.m. 4 a.m. 8 a.m. 12 p.m. 4 p.m.

Delayed sleep-wake phase disorder

Advanced sleep-wake phase disorder

Normal sleep

Irregular sleep-wake rhythm disorder

Non-24-hour sleep-wake rhythm disorder

FIGURE 7-1: Circadian rhythm phases and associated disorders.

You can experience circadian rhythm sleep-wake disorders that don't fit with the classifications I describe in this section. And they may have symptoms not otherwise specified in the classifications.

Researchers suspect that the *suprachiasmatic nucleus*, which is the circadian pacemaker, somehow malfunctions in some individuals and causes circadian rhythm sleep-wake disorders. I talk more about the suprachiasmatic nucleus in Chapter 4.

TECHNICAL STUFF

Getting diagnosed with a circadian rhythm sleep-wake disorder

When you see your healthcare provider for a suspected circadian rhythm sleep-wake disorder, they look at your history and may ask for sleep logs (see Chapter 9) accompanied by actigraphy data whenever possible (see Chapter 10) for 7–14 days to understand your sleep patterns. Each disorder's diagnosis is based on criteria from the American Academy of Sleep Medicine's International Classification of Sleep Disorders. These criteria consist of the specific symptoms for each disorder I describe in the earlier "Recognizing symptoms of circadian rhythm disorders" section as well as the points in the following discussions.

REMEMBER

The diagnostic criteria for each sleep disorder specifies that specialists cannot better explain the identified sleep disturbance by another current sleep disorder, medical or neurological disorder, mental disorder, and medication or substance use disorder.

Delayed sleep-wake phase disorder

If your sleep logs and actigraphy show that you're experiencing a delay in the timing of your usual sleep period, your specialist may diagnose delayed sleep-wake phase disorder. Specialists consider this disorder problematic only when the patient is past adolescence or young adulthood because most adolescents and young adults prefer to go to sleep late and get up later. As long as the sleep doesn't interfere regularly with commitments or daily life, young people can safely go to sleep and wake up late.

Advanced sleep-wake phase disorder

If your sleep logs and actigraphy show that your major sleep period is significantly advanced, which means you fall asleep significantly earlier and awaken earlier than usual, your specialist may diagnose you with advanced sleep phase disorder.

TIP

Don't let age automatically rule you in or out. Advanced sleep-wake phase disorder is most common among elderly individuals, but the disorder can also affect younger individuals as well.

Irregular sleep-wake rhythm disorder

If your sleep logs and actigraphy show that you have no clear sleep-wake circadian pattern and at least three multiple irregular sleep bouts within a 24-hour period, your specialist may diagnose you with irregular sleep-wake rhythm disorder. This disorder usually implies involvement of the brain, and it can sometimes tie into a neurological disorder. For example, a person might have a neurodegenerative disorder, such as dementia, or a child might have a developmental disorder.

Non-24-hour sleep-wake rhythm disorder

If your sleep logs and actigraphy show that for at least 14 days, your sleep-wake times experience a delay (or advance) each day that makes your circadian period usually longer than 24 hours, your specialist may diagnose you with non-24-hour sleep-wake rhythm disorder. In this condition, your internal circadian pacemaker doesn't follow the 24-hour light-dark cycle.

Many individuals who have this disorder are non-sighted individuals because they don't receive the photic or light input, which means they can't adapt to the environmental cue of the light and dark cycle. As Nathaniel Kleitman (the grandfather of sleep science) in his 1938 Mammoth Cave experiments and Max Plack Institute for Behavioral Physiology researchers in their 1966 bunker study found, individuals in totally dark environments, showed that without external cues, they engage in what's called *free-running*, meaning they revert to their natural cycle, which in most people is more than 24 hours — about 24.6 hours. And so, with each successive night, they want to sleep a little later and get up a little later. Individuals with non-24-hour sleep-wake rhythm disorder start free-running because they don't have that photic input.

Shift work disorder

If your sleep logs and actigraphy show that you have a disturbed sleep and wake pattern and you have rotating, night, or early morning shifts, your specialist may diagnose you with shift work disorder.

Jet lag disorder

If your sleep logs and actigraphy show that you have impaired daytime functioning, general malaise, and general body system problems — such as gastrointestinal disturbances that occur within a day or two after your arrival at your destination — your specialist may diagnose you with jet lag disorder.

TIP

Since most individuals have an internal clock with a period of longer than 24 hours, westward travel is often easier than eastward travel, as described in more detail in the next section.

Receiving treatment for a circadian rhythm sleep-wake disorder

Each of these circadian rhythm sleep-wake disorders stems from disruptions in the circadian rhythm, and understanding your own pattern is the key to finding the right treatment approach. Managing a circadian rhythm sleep-wake disorder is a collaborative process between you and your healthcare provider.

Delayed sleep phase disorder and advanced sleep phase disorder

Treatment for delayed or advanced sleep-wake phase disorders often includes light therapy and melatonin. Regarding light therapy, your doctor may

>> **Instruct you to use bright light therapy** in the morning for delayed sleep-wake phase disorder or in the evening for advanced sleep-wake phase disorder to help reset your internal clock.

>> **Recommend that you go outside to get natural light** within five minutes of waking up, but if you're awake before sunrise, you might consider obtaining a light box. You can receive 10,000 *lux* (the measurement of light intensity for a given area) for at least half an hour from the light to help synchronize your internal clock.

Conversely, within about two hours before bedtime, you should have only dim light. By *dim*, I mean that you should allow yourself just enough light to identify objects, so that you don't bump into anything in your environment.

You might also find relief by taking melatonin in low doses — tailored to your specific needs and based on your healthcare provider's consultation — to aid the process of shifting rhythms. For example, instead of the typical five to ten milligrams of melatonin people usually take, your sleep specialist might recommend 0.5 milligrams or less about an hour before your desired bedtime.

TIP

Communicate with your doctor to let them know how the melatonin dose works for you. You might have to adjust it a few times to find the right amount and correct timing.

You can also consider seeking help from a behavioral sleep medicine or CBT-I specialist to help with these disorders. Refer to Table 7-1 for more about cognitive behavioral therapies.

Irregular sleep-wake rhythm disorder

This challenging disorder is difficult to treat because sleep periods are scattered over the 24-hour period. Having irregular sleep-wake rhythm disorder is truly challenging for children in school and adults at work because they can get sleepy at very different times and their sleep is fragmented. Visiting a sleep center to see a sleep specialist is important to help you manage this condition.

Non-24-hour sleep-wake rhythm disorder

If you suffer from the challenging non-24-hour sleep-wake rhythm disorder, you can benefit from a sleep specialist's management. In addition to treatment from a psychologist who has expertise in behavioral sleep medicine, a sleep specialist might prescribe *tasimelteon*, which is the only FDA-approved medication to treat this specific circadian rhythm sleep-wake disorder.

Shift work disorder

While there is no perfect solution — especially if you have rotating shifts — your sleep specialist can recommend behavioral treatments such as

>> Getting bright light therapy and taking melatonin, which may help adjust your sleep patterns when you're starting a shift.

>> Maintaining good *sleep hygiene* (optimizing your sleep environment and sleep-related behavior) so you can avoid naps that might disrupt your sleep-wake schedule.

>> If you can't fall asleep or return to sleep within about 20 minutes, engaging in a drowsy activity in another room, then returning to bed.

>> Keeping your sleeping environment soundproof and lightproof.

>> Avoiding clock-watching.

TIP

If you struggle to sleep or stay awake as needed, you can ask your sleep specialists about medications (for the short-term), such as hypnotics like zolpidem or stimulants like modafinil and armodafinil.

Jet lag disorder

Similar to shift work disorder, jet lag disorder takes adjustments. You can try to acclimate to the destination time zone by gradually adjusting your sleep and wake times. However, changing your sleep schedule isn't always feasible, and you may need to use the behavioral methods I outline in the preceding section "Shift work disorder."

Eastward travel often leads to difficulty with sleep onset because it aligns with an earlier internal circadian time. Conversely, westward travel can cause evening sleepiness and fatigue, aligning with the traveler's internal clock, which promotes sleep. Traveling westward is generally easier because the natural tendency is to want to sleep a little later and get up later, fitting with the average internal circadian clock of 24.6 hours. This tendency aligns with the typical experience where it's easier to adjust to sleeping later rather than earlier (for example, when traveling eastward).

WARNING

Medications such as mild hypnotics or stimulants may be beneficial, but you must test medications before the trip to avoid being overly sedated. (And be aware of dangers and cautions around mixing sedative medications with alcohol.) You don't want to sleep through a flight so deeply that you don't realize it's time to get off the plane — or be sedated by the side effects that can linger and impact performance during your first days at your journey's destination!

IN THIS CHAPTER

» Investigating the challenges of poor breathing while asleep

» Scratching beneath the surface of sleep-related movement disorders

» Peeling back the layers of parasomnias

Chapter **8**

Exploring Sleep Disorders of the Active Kind

Whether you're an adult or a child, you can experience a number of sleep disorders that involve physical aspects of your sleep habits. For example, you question whether you should seek a doctor's help when you notice your bedpartner gasping to breathe while asleep, you need to get up and move your legs every time you go to sleep, or your child suddenly screams in the middle of the night several times a week.

This chapter offers information about the active type of sleep disorders, from how to identify symptoms and possible causes of various conditions such as sleep apnea, restless legs syndrome, and sleepwalking to seeking treatment.

Breathing That Changes When You Sleep

Sleep-related breathing disorders encompass several conditions that affect adults and children, including obstructive sleep apnea (OSA) and a variety of different central sleep apnea syndromes. They also include *sleep-related hypoventilation syndromes* (in which you can't breathe deeply or quickly enough) and *hypoxemia disorders* (which can result in life-threatening low levels of oxygen in the blood).

You can also experience isolated symptoms and normal variants of snoring and sleep-related groaning (*catathrenia*) — although medical research has mixed conclusions about the clinical significance and consequences of these occurrences.

In this section, I focus on the main disorder — obstructive sleep apnea — and sprinkle material about the others throughout the discussion.

Recognizing the scope of sleep apnea

Obstructive sleep apnea (OSA) is a very common condition that affects about 24 percent of men and about 9 percent of women between the ages of 30 and 60. After the age of 60, OSA becomes more prevalent. In kids, about 3 percent of the population has obstructive sleep apnea.

REMEMBER

For children, the problems with breathing during sleep are frequently missed, and the 3-percent figure may be an underestimation. Considering a child's anatomical features that may influence the continued development of the airway is important. These features may increase the risk of developing OSA that occurs with greater percentages in adults.

WARNING

Obstructive sleep apnea can have a number of serious consequences and negative impacts on people's health, including

>> **Higher risk for cardiovascular diseases:** because the data from the Sleep Heart Health Study — a National Heart, Lung, and Blood Institute-sponsored project — suggests that people with obstructive sleep apnea have 138 percent higher odds of heart failure, 58 percent higher odds of stroke, and 27 percent higher odds of coronary heart disease than those without OSA

>> **A higher accident risk** because of falling asleep during activities such as driving or operating heavy machinery

>> **A reduced ability to concentrate, focus, remember, stay awake, and perform tasks** that require higher executive function (such as driving, again)

>> **The risk of experiencing or worsening mental disorders** such as anxiety and depression

Obstructive sleep apnea is often worse during the REM (rapid eye movement) stage of sleep — when dreaming happens, your muscles are limp, and your brain is active — because your breathing normally becomes shallow and irregular and your heart rate can become irregular, even if you are otherwise healthy. See Appendix B for a look at sleep study measurements that indicate various aspects of obstructive sleep apnea.

Exploring causes of sleep apnea

Many reasons can underlie why someone might have OSA. Sleep specialists group these reasons into categories of characteristics called *endotypes*:

>> **Anatomical:** When someone's airway is more likely to be blocked while sleeping due to a structural issue like large tonsils or a small jaw.

>> **Fluid shift:** When fluid shifts from the legs to the neck when someone is lying down, creating pressure around their throat, making it hard for them to breathe. People who have high blood pressure, heart failure, or end-stage kidney failure often experience this shift.

>> **High loop gain:** When the breathing control system becomes unstable resulting in recurrent pauses in breathing during sleep.

These recurrent breathing pauses happen when someone has other medical conditions (for example, serious heart or kidney problems). The system controlling breathing during sleep is on high alert and is quite sensitive to the physical stress caused by the other medical conditions. This sensitivity affects the system's ability to manage and maintain blood gas levels (blood oxygen saturation and carbon dioxide), resulting in sleep apnea.

>> **Low arousal threshold:** When people wake up too easily from sleep, resulting in disruption in their sleep-related breathing. Up to a third of all people with obstructive sleep apnea have this endotype.

REMEMBER

Waking up is the brain's response to problems with breathing and is an important survival mechanism. If such awakenings happen repetitively, the job that sleep is trying to do is disrupted and the result is sleepiness, grogginess, irritability, and possible complaint of insomnia.

>> **Reduced lung volume:** When low lung volume makes it harder for people to fully inflate their chest, which can promote upper airway collapse. Physicians see reduced lung volume in patients who experience these problems because of some underlying lung disease.

>> **Poor muscle function:** When the muscles that keep the airway open — like the *genioglossus*, which is the primary tongue muscle — don't work properly, especially during sleep. Many muscles of the upper airway, face, tongue, and mouth can influence and be influenced by the activity of breathing.

Everyone who has OSA is unique and may have a mix of these endotypes. However, these endotypes are integral to understanding the causes of obstructive sleep apnea and, in the future, will undoubtedly help doctors and sleep specialists develop targeted treatment for these endotypes.

In addition to the endotypes, you find other factors that can increase your risk for having obstructive sleep apnea, such as

>> Family history of sleep apnea

>> Alcohol consumption

>> Smoking

>> Use of sedatives

>> Nasal congestion or deviated septum

>> Menopause

>> Endocrine disorders (such as thyroid disease)

>> Obesity

REMEMBER

Obesity is the most common risk factor for sleep apnea, and roughly 30 to 70 percent of the people who have obstructive sleep apnea are overweight (defined by a body mass index of 25 or greater).

In terms of sex, women tend to have less severe and less frequent apneas during the night than men. However, after menopause, the prevalence rates of obstructive sleep apnea in post-menopausal women can get very close to that of men. Doctors don't fully understand the reasons for the increased prevalence rates, although they believe that the upper airway is sensitive to estrogen and progesterone. If women undergo hormone replacement therapy (HRT), then their risk decreases to pre-menopausal levels.

Recognizing symptoms of sleep apnea

If you suspect that you might have obstructive sleep apnea, look for the primary and secondary symptoms, as outlined in Table 8-1.

TABLE 8-1   **Symptoms of Obstructive Sleep Apnea**

Primary Symptoms	Secondary Symptoms
Loud, disruptive snoring	Cold hands and feet; sweating at night
Breathing pauses that someone else witnesses	Holding your breath, gasping, or choking while you sleep
Excessive daytime sleepiness	Not feeling refreshed or having headaches upon awakening (from nighttime sleep or naps)

Getting diagnosed with sleep apnea

If you experience any of the symptoms you find in the preceding section on a regular basis, make an appointment with your primary care physician and ask for a referral to a sleep specialist (see more on how to get a referral in Chapter 9). When you visit a sleep specialist, they examine and evaluate many aspects of your physical condition and symptoms, including

>> **Your nighttime sleep habits and your daytime sleepiness.** Sleep specialists often evaluate daytime sleepiness by using the Epworth Sleepiness scale, which I discuss more in Chapter 9.

>> **Your age, body mass index (BMI), neck size, and sex.** If you're older than 50, have a neck size that's greater than 40 cm, and you're a male, you are more predisposed to having obstructive sleep apnea than others.

>> **Your responses on the STOP-BANG screening questionnaire for obstructive sleep apnea.** This questionnaire, developed by Dr. Frances Chung at the University of Toronto, asks a series of yes/no questions that focus on key symptoms and risk factors. You can find versions of the STOP-BANG questionnaire online, for example, on the website of the Ohio Sleep Medicine Institute at www.sleepmedicine.com. The following mini-table shows what the letters of the acronym stand for and the related questions.

The letters	The questions
S for Snoring	Do you snore loudly enough to disturb your bedpartner or to be heard beyond a closed door?
T for Tired	Do you often feel tired, fatigued, or sleepy?
O for Observed	Has anyone observed you stop breathing or gasping or choking during sleep?
P for Pressure	Do you have high blood pressure?
B for Body mass index	Do you have a high body mass index?
A for Age	Are you older than 50?
N for Neck size	Is your neck large?
G for Gender (sex)	Are you male?

Screening adults for sleep apnea

Your sleep specialist also conducts two phases of screening. In the first phase, they look to see whether you experience at least one of these conditions:

Habitual snoring, having interruptions in your breathing, or both during sleep

Holding your breath as you wake up, gasping, or choking

Sleepiness, fatigue, insomnia, or other symptoms leading to decreased sleep-related quality of life

If you experience one of these conditions, your sleep specialist moves onto the next diagnostic phase and orders a laboratory or home sleep study for you (see more in Chapter 9 about how sleep studies work). Your sleep specialist reviews your in-lab or in-home sleep study data to see whether you experience five or more incidents that are called *predominantly obstructive abnormal breathing events* per hour of sleep in a lab or per hour of monitoring at home.

TECHNICAL STUFF

ABNORMAL BREATHING EVENTS

Predominantly obstructive abnormal breathing falls into several categories:

- **Obstructive apneas,** where you have pauses in breathing that last at least 10 seconds

- **Hypopneas,** where you experience decreases in airflow that also last 10 seconds or more, and you also have a decrease in oxygen saturation or have a brief awakening

- **Respiratory effort-related arousals,** which is when you have to work harder to breathe, and that extra effort results in an awakening

In addition to these obstructive events, there are also *central events*, which happen when your diaphragm pauses for at least 10 seconds. Then there is *mixed apnea*, which is a combination of obstructive and central events.

If you have mainly central events (five or more of these events per hour) on the in-lab or home monitoring and have symptoms similar to those of obstructive sleep apnea but without snoring, your sleep specialist may diagnose you with one of the syndromes of central sleep apnea.

Central sleep apnea in adults, children, and infants is less common than obstructive sleep apnea, and the diagnosis of these syndromes is based on

- The presence of specific medical disorders (e.g., atrial fibrillation/flutter, congestive heart failure)

- Neurologic disorders

- Circumstances (for example, high altitude, prematurity, use of positive airway pressure device)

- Medications (for example, opioid or other respiratory depressant)

- Cheyne-Stokes breathing (i.e., a repetitive pattern of fast, deep breathing that decreases to an apnea)

- Sleep-related hypoventilation disorders in which breathing is slow or shallow, and the partial pressure of carbon dioxide ($PaCO_2$) — which is the amount of carbon dioxide in your blood and how well carbon dioxide can move out of your body — is noninvasively measured during a sleep study. This measure — combined with obesity, certain genetic mutations, neural tumors, lung or airway conditions, neurological or muscle disorders, and medications — determines the diagnosis of a specific central sleep apnea syndrome. Lastly, sleep-related hypoxemia disorders are diagnosed by decreases in oxygen content of 88 percent or less in adults or 90 percent or less in children during sleep for five minutes or more. The oxygen desaturations are not fully explained by sleep-related hypoventilation, obstructive sleep apnea, or other sleep-related breathing disorder.

REMEMBER

You must have five or more abnormal breathing events per hour of sleep to be diagnosed with OSA (if you have the symptoms, including sleepiness). If you don't have the symptoms, you must have 15 events or more per hour. Fewer than 5 events per hour is considered normal, 5 to 14.9 events per hour is mild, 15 to 30 events per hour is considered moderate, and 30 events or more per hour is considered severe.

Screening children for sleep apnea

For kids to receive an obstructive sleep apnea diagnosis, they must experience one or more of these symptoms:

Snoring

Labored, paradoxical *thoracoabdominal* (for example, a condition where the chest and abdomen don't work in synchrony when the child breathes), or obstructed breathing during sleep

Sleepiness, hyperactivity, behavioral problems, or learning and other cognitive problems

TIP

Often, sleep-disordered breathing or obstructive sleep apnea in kids can closely mimic the symptoms of attention-deficit hyperactivity disorder (ADHD). If your child experiences ADHD-like symptoms, ask your pediatrician to order a sleep test or provide a referral to a sleep specialist to make sure that they don't have a sleep disordered breathing component.

With kids, at-home sleep studies aren't currently recommended for the diagnosis of sleep apnea, so if your child needs a study, you go to the laboratory. To diagnose a child with obstructive sleep apnea, during the sleep study the specialist looks for one or more of the same events that they look for in adults. (See the sidebar "Abnormal breathing events" also in this chapter.)

If your child is symptomatic (see the symptoms listed earlier in this section), experiences one or more abnormal breathing event per hour in the sleep study, and/or has decreased breathing rate with increased carbon dioxide levels in association with either snoring, flattening of the breathing pattern in inspiration, and/or paradoxical thoracoabdominal motion, the doctor will likely diagnose your child with obstructive sleep apnea, providing the symptoms are not better explained by another current disorder, medication, or substance use. Diagnosing and treating children who are symptomatic and have OSA is important because delayed growth can be a consequence of untreated sleep apnea.

Receiving treatment for sleep apnea

The three main treatments for obstructive sleep apnea include

>> **Positive airway pressure treatment (PAP):** The patient uses a machine that delivers air pressure through a mask they wear over their nose, or both their nose and mouth, during sleep. The air pressure helps to keep their airways open.

REMEMBER

The PAP machine masks come in many varieties and sizes; see Figure 8-1 for a look at the one PAP device (AirSense 11 CPAP machine) as presented on the ResMed website under CPAP machines (www.resmed.com/en-us/sleep-apnea/cpap-products/cpap-machines). Proper mask fitting and comfort are the most important aspects of the whole PAP treatment approach. See Figure 8-2, also found on the ResMed website. Paying attention to detail regarding mask fitting translates to a better experience for the patient, better comfort, and more consistent use of the treatment.

You find two main types of PAP machines, which automatically deliver air pressure (within prescribed ranges) that increases and decreases during the night to provide the lowest pressure necessary to keep the upper airway open:

- *Continuous positive airway pressure (CPAP)*, which sends a stream of continuous air pressure into the person's airway.
- *Bilevel positive airway pressure (BPAP)*, which gives the person more pressure as they breathe in, and less pressure when they breathe out.

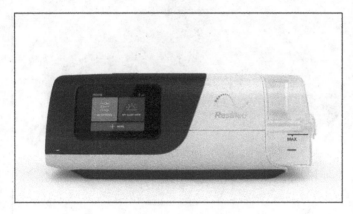

FIGURE 8-1:
An AirSense 11 CPAP machine.

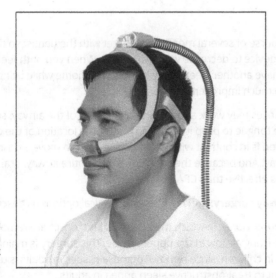

FIGURE 8-2:
Getting a comfortable fit for a CPAP mask.

>> **Oral appliances:** These prescribed mouthguards or retainers move the patient's lower jaw forward by clipping onto your upper and lower teeth and using hinges or tabs that prevent your lower jaw from being pushed backwards and/or expand the roof of the mouth to decrease symptoms. For example, see the Vivos mRNA appliance in Figure 8-3, as shown on the Vivos website (https://vivos.com).

If your doctor prescribes an oral appliance, a dentist with sleep apnea experience takes molds of your upper and lower teeth, sends the molds out to have your device made, and then sees you again to fit you with that device.

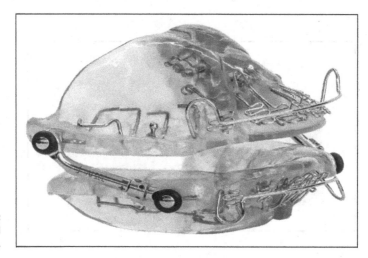

FIGURE 8-3:
A Vivos oral appliance.

Over the course of several months, you meet with the dentist so that they can adjust the device to decrease your symptoms. When you both feel the fit is right, you have another sleep study in a lab or at home while using the device to see how much improvement you have.

WARNING

Oral appliances may work at one particular region of the airway, such as the base of the tongue to prop it open, (no matter the location of the obstruction). This situation is in contrast with PAP machines, which move air through your entire airway. And because they don't open the entire airway, oral appliances may be less effective than CPAP.

>> **Upper airway surgery:** You have several surgical options as described here:

- *Adenotonsillectomy,* in which the adenoids and tonsils are removed if they are restricting airflow in the upper airway. This surgery is mainly performed in children, since removal of these tissues in adults is usually not sufficient to treat obstructive sleep apnea in adults.

- *Uvulopalatopharyngoplasty,* in which surgeons remove some of the soft tissue in the back of the airway to create more space for the airway.

- *Maxillomandibular advancement* (MMA), which consists of advancing the upper and lower jaws forward to create more space to open up the airway.

- *Hypoglossal nerve stimulation,* which requires a surgeon to implant an electrode onto the hypoglossal nerve in the *genioglossus* (the major tongue muscle) and run the electrode wire underneath the skin to a pacemaker-like device in the chest wall. The electrode provides a small electric shock (not enough to wake you up) to move your tongue forward and keep your upper airway open.

TIP

Using CPAPs, BPAPs, or oral appliances, or having upper airway surgery can help improve your overall quality of life by not only reducing the severity of obstructive sleep apnea, but also reducing high blood pressure!

Supplemental therapies that can help with sleep apnea

In addition to the three main therapies, your sleep specialist may also recommend

>> **A weight-loss regimen,** which can also reduce the size of the fat pads on either side of the upper airway, allowing the airway to properly open.

REMEMBER

Doctors consider weight loss an *adjunctive therapy* (or supplemental therapy) because in most cases, it can't cure a patient with OSA, but can reduce the severity. However, weight loss is a powerful tool for the management of sleep-related breathing disorders. Researchers show that a change in body weight by 10 percent can have a significant impact. Also, the FDA has recently (as of this writing) approved a weight loss medication, Zepbound (tirzepatide), for the treatment of obstructive sleep apnea and obesity. So weight loss will become an important treatment for obstructive sleep apnea in the future.

>> **Behavioral modification therapy (BMT),** which helps patients manage obstructive sleep apnea by sleeping on their side instead of their back. As many as 60 percent of patients who have obstructive sleep apnea experience their condition when they're on their back in the supine position (or it worsens in that position), so getting them off their back is helpful.

Some people can adjust their sleep position without help, and others need extra help from devices that can either detect body position and notify them when they're on their back or use cushions or apparel that prevent them from sleeping on their back. Other patients benefit by sleeping on an inclined cushion (an incline of about 30 degrees) instead of lying flat on their backs.

TIP

If you need help staying on your side to sleep and aren't ready to invest in a consumer product, try using full body pillows, or just propping yourself on your side with extra regular-sized pillows. It's not a perfect solution if you move around a lot in your sleep, but it's worth a shot.

Treatments for specific sleep apnea endotypes

Sleep specialists may try a few other treatments for specific obstructive sleep apnea *endotypes* (subtypes of the disease):

>> **Rostral fluid shift:** Your doctor may prescribe diuretics to reduce the fluid in your body, and may also have you sleep with your head tilted up, typically more than 30 degrees to decrease the chance of this fluid shift towards your head.

>> **Lung volume:** Technically, doctors can't increase lung volume, but they've found that when they apply negative pressure to the outside of the chest wall by using a *chest cuirass* (a rigid shell) and *wrap-type system* (nylon poncho around a semicylindrical tent-like support), they can actually reduce the area resistance in the upper airway. In doing so, they can open up the upper airway.

>> **High loop gain:** Supplemental oxygen and *acetazolamide*, which is a respiratory stimulant medication, can help to reduce *loop gain* (instability of the breathing control system) when the specialist recognizes that the loop gain is too high.

>> **Low arousal threshold:** Some people have low arousal thresholds, which means that they wake up easily. In this case, increasing the threshold by up to 30 percent with sedatives can have a corresponding decrease in the severity of obstructive sleep apnea for those with this endotype.

Moving Excessively in Your Sleep: Sleep-Related Movement Disorders

Sleep-related movement disorders are conditions that cause you to involuntarily move during sleep, which disrupts sleep and can lead to daytime fatigue or sleepiness. The most common of these disorders include

>> **Restless legs syndrome (RLS),** which happens when you have an irresistible urge to move your legs (and even arms) while awake

>> **Periodic limb movement disorder (PLMD),** which happens when you periodically (every few seconds) move your limbs while you sleep

>> **Rhythmic movement disorders,** such as head banging or rocking, occur during sleep — especially at sleep onset in children

RLS is common, affecting approximately 5 to 10 percent of the population. Doctors don't know much about the exact cause of RLS, but they think it may be linked to how the brain regulates movement through pathways that involve the neurotransmitter dopamine. Factors that may contribute to RLS include

>> Genetics, iron deficiency, and certain medications with toxins often being culprits.

>> Underlying medical conditions, such as pregnancy, diabetes, kidney disease, and peripheral neuropathy, are also associated with RLS.

RLS triggers can vary but may include substances such as alcohol, caffeine, and nicotine, especially when consumed before rest or bedtime.

Recognizing movement disorder symptoms

The symptoms of RLS are

>> Having a terrible urge to move your legs that worsens with rest and near bedtime, but temporarily improves with activity like walking or stretching

>> Worsening symptoms in confined spaces such as airplane seats or restaurant booths, leading to a need to move around

>> Uncomfortable sensations that feel like crawling, itching, pulling, or throbbing that generally feel like they are deep within your legs

>> Sensations that happen in your arms or other parts of the body and usually occur on both sides

If you have PLMD, you won't usually be aware of its symptoms; instead, someone else usually observes the symptoms, which include

>> Repetitive kicking or twitching of the legs or arms during sleep, typically every 20 to 40 seconds, sometimes throughout the night.

>> Movements that occasionally wake you up, but are more commonly disruptive to bed partners. Many times, couples sleep in separate bedrooms if one person has symptoms of this disorder but has not sought medical help.

>> Daytime fatigue or sleepiness, resulting from disturbed sleep patterns.

TIP

The easiest way to distinguish between RLS and PLMD is that RLS patients are awake during episodes, whereas PLMD occurs during sleep. And many patients suffer from both RLS and PLMD.

Getting a movement disorder diagnosis

Your doctor can give you an RLS diagnosis primarily through reviewing your patient history and exam. They must see that these symptoms cause significant distress or impairment in various aspects of your life and that the condition is not due to other disorders, such as medical, neurologic, sleep, or behavioral conditions.

On the other hand, a PLMD diagnosis requires an examination and in-lab sleep study typically after your bedpartner reports that you frequently move your limbs during sleep, and that it causes sleep disturbance or impaired functioning.

REMEMBER

You are often not aware that you have PLMD because you're most likely asleep when symptoms occur.

An in-lab sleep study records limb movements and checks for a pattern of movements at a certain frequency, interval, and amplitude, and the frequency in which they are associated with brief awakenings (arousals) from sleep. Sleep lab professionals look for these elements to diagnose PLMD:

- Movements that are 0.5 to 10 seconds in duration, and are separated by at least 5 seconds to 90 seconds

- At least four limb movements that meet the timing criteria count as one episode of periodic limb movement

- Greater than 15 episodes of periodic limb movements per hour for adults, and greater than 5 per hour for children

And the other criterion for a PLMD diagnosis is that the condition has to cause a clinically significant sleep disturbance or impairment in an important area of functioning — such as mental, physical, social, occupational, educational, or behavioral — and the symptoms are not better explained by another disorder.

TIP

Eighty percent of RLS patients also exhibit PLMS, but the rate of occurrence of PLMS in the general population is unknown. Doctors see PLMS occur about 30 percent of the time when they are doing sleep studies on patients for other conditions. (See Appendix B for a sleep study measurement showing a patient that has PLMS.)

Receiving treatment for RLS or PLMD

To treat either or both restless legs syndrome and periodic limb movement disorder, your specialist may prescribe one or more of four classes of medications:

>> **Dopaminergic agents:** Medications such as ropinirole (Requip), pramipexole (Mirapex), and rotigotine (Neupro), are often used to treat these conditions. This type of medication can be effective, but it also carries a risk of *augmentation* (an increase in symptom severity, earlier onset, or spread to other limbs). Augmentation can happen at any time — from a week to years after starting the medication — and increasing the dosage can actually worsen the condition.

>> **Benzodiazepines:** Mild tranquilizers, such as clonazepam (Klonopin), similar to those used for parasomnias (see the section "Walking and Screaming in Your Sleep: Parasomnias" later in this chapter), can also be effective. However, the exact mechanism of how tranquilizers work on RLS or PLMD is unclear. Sleep specialists believe that these medications increase the arousal threshold, making the patient less aware of movements.

>> **Anticonvulsants/pain medications:** Gabapentin (Neurontin) and pregabalin (Lyrica), are common choices for treatment. Doctors like them because they not only treat the RLS and PLMD but also enhance sleep quality by increasing deep sleep and reducing the time required to fall asleep.

>> **Opiates:** These medications can be very effective but must be prescribed with caution due to the risks of dependence, tolerance, and respiratory suppression, which could lead to central apnea or other breathing issues during sleep (especially if taken with alcohol).

WARNING

Due to the potential side effects and the complex nature of these movement sleep disorders, always follow your doctor's instructions *exactly* if they prescribe opiates for you to treat RLS or PLMD.

Your doctor may also recommend a *ferritin-level test* and other iron tests because iron deficiency can result in these disorders and supplemental iron can effectively treat these conditions in iron-deficient individuals. Taking medications such as antidepressants is also associated with these disorders.

Other sleep-related movement disorders

Some sleep-related movement disorders are relatively minor and common among people, but are still worth seeking help for if you can't sleep.

Nocturnal muscle cramps

Nocturnal muscle cramps, also known as *charley horses*, involve a painful sensation in a muscle associated with sudden, involuntary muscle hardness or tightness.

This occurs due to strong muscle contractions, often while in bed, arising during either wakefulness or sleep.

Nocturnal muscle cramps are a common condition, but doctors don't always know its exact cause; sometimes cramps may be linked to a patient's electrolyte imbalances (for example, they may have low potassium). Unfortunately, no definitive treatments exist, but short-term muscle relaxants or analgesic medication may provide some relief.

You can sometimes get relief if you forcefully stretch your affected muscles.

Sleep-related bruxism

Your doctor may diagnose you with sleep-related *bruxism* (tooth grinding or clenching) if you experience repetitive jaw muscle activity characterized by tooth grinding or clenching during sleep, along with one or more clinical signs:

Abnormal tooth wear

Transient morning jaw muscle pain or fatigue

Temporal headache

Usually, a dentist or a bedpartner notices this condition first. A doctor doesn't usually conduct a sleep study unless the bruxism is frequent. In this case, they conduct these tests to rule out conditions such as seizure disorders.

Treatment options are limited, but you can try muscle relaxants and oral appliances like mouthguards to prevent teeth damage. In recent years, sleep specialists have begun to consider psychological disturbances, especially anxiety disorders, to be potential underlying factors, and often refer patients to psychologists for stress management when their bruxism is severe. Ruling out the presence of a sleep-related breathing disorder that may be occurring along with bruxism is also important.

Sleep-related rhythmic movement disorder

When you experience sleep-related rhythmic movement disorder, you may find yourself making repetitive, rhythmical movements that involve large muscles, like those in your head, torso, arms, and legs. These movements are semi-voluntary, meaning you might not be fully aware that you're doing them, especially if they occur as you're falling asleep or while you're asleep.

These movements predominantly occur just as you're falling asleep at night, but you can also experience them during naps or when you're drowsy or asleep. The condition may interfere with your normal sleep, impair your daytime functioning, or cause self-inflicted bodily injury if you don't take preventive measures. Common movements include body rocking, headbanging, or head rolling, sometimes resulting in associated headaches.

TIP

A sleep specialist may order a sleep study to ensure a proper diagnosis. You may find some relief by seeking psychotherapy, but successful treatment by psychotherapy may not be consistent. Benzodiazepines, such as clonazepam, or relaxation techniques may also help.

Unspecified sleep-related movement disorders

An unspecified sleep-related movement disorder category exists for conditions that don't fit into other classifications. Neurologists often help sleep specialists diagnose these rarer conditions through sleep studies:

>> **Benign sleep myoclonus of infancy** is when infants experience repetitive jerks of the limbs, trunk, or their entire bodies during sleep.

>> **Propriospinal myoclonus at sleep onset happens when adults experience sudden jerks that** mainly affect the abdomen, trunk, and neck near bedtime.

>> **Isolated sleep-related movement symptoms and normal variants** that are benign include

- *Excessive fragmentary myoclonus,* in which brief, small movements happen at the corners of the mouth, fingers, or toes, or — without any visible movement at all — are noted incidentally on the PSG (see Chapter 10).

- *Hypnagogic foot tremor,* in which the feet or toes rhythmically move for a few seconds to minutes during the transition between wake and sleep, or during light NREM N1 and N2 sleep.

- *Alternating leg muscle activation,* in which the leg muscle (the anterior tibialis) is briefly activated in one leg in alternation with similar activation in the other leg during sleep or arousals from sleep.

- *Sleep starts or hypnic jerks,* in which you feel a sudden full-body jerk and often a sensation of falling. This phenomenon may be due to a momentary lapse in the normal inhibition of spinal motor neurons during sleep. While benign, persistent issues may warrant psychotherapy, with image rehearsal therapy being an option if nightmares or the sensation of falling are problematic.

Walking and Screaming in Your Sleep: Parasomnias

Parasomnias are disruptive sleep disorders that specialists categorize into four major groups via the American Academy of Sleep Medicine's International Classification of Sleep Disorders: NREM-related parasomnias, REM-related parasomnias, other parasomnias, and isolated symptoms and normal variants.

The category of isolated symptoms and normal variants can include benign behaviors, such as sleep talking. I cover the other, more disruptive categories in the following sections.

NREM-related parasomnias

NREM-related parasomnias are disorders of arousal (awakenings) from NREM sleep that are usual brief (but may last as long as 30-40 minutes) and include

>> **Confusional arousals:** This is mental confusion or confused behavior upon waking, from deep NREM sleep, with episodes sometimes lasting several minutes.

>> **Sleepwalking (*somnambulism*):** This happens when a person walks or performs complex behaviors while asleep and doesn't remember the events afterwards. More than a third of children may experience sleepwalking at some point, and genetic factors appear to play a role in all disorders related to arousal from NREM sleep, but particularly in sleepwalking. The rate of childhood sleepwalking increases with the number of affected parents: 22 percent of children might sleepwalk if neither parent has experienced sleepwalking, 45 percent if one parent is affected, and 60 percent when both are affected.

WARNING

Don't awaken someone who is sleepwalking because they may be disoriented or react unpredictably. A 2013 report on a French sleep study (available on the PubMed website at https://pubmed.ncbi.nlm.nih.gov/23450499) showed that, close to 60 percent of sleepwalkers reported violent sleep-related behaviors toward themselves or their bedpartners, including injuries that required medical care for at least one episode in 17 percent.

>> **Sleep terrors (night terrors):** Episodes of screaming, intense fear, and flailing while still asleep with no recollection afterwards and the individual may be inconsolable during the event.

REMEMBER

Sleepwalking and sleep terrors often occur together in children. It is common for a child to experience both disorders, sometimes starting with sleep terrors and then sleepwalking, or vice versa.

>> **Sleep-related eating disorder:** Engaging in eating behaviors while asleep with no memory of the activity.

>> **Sleep-related abnormal sexual behaviors or sexsomnia:** Sexual behavior (for example, masturbation, fondling, sexual intercourse) that occurs during sleep. These behaviors are classified as a subtype of NREM-related parasomnias, and just like other NREM-related parasomnias, the person has no recall of the occurrence of these episodes. Often the person's bedpartner is surprised or shocked by the occurrence, but when they confront the individual the next day, they find that the person has no recollection of the behavior.

As the American Academy of Sleep Medicine's International Classification of Sleep Disorders establishes, NREM-related parasomnias typically share several common features that comprise the diagnostic criteria for these disorders:

They occur during incomplete awakenings from sleep.

The patient may have limited or inappropriate responsiveness to others.

They often include minimal cognitive activity or dream imagery.

Patients might have partial or full amnesia of the event.

They can't be explained by other disorders or substance use.

REM-related parasomnias

REM-related parasomnias occur during REM sleep and include

>> **REM sleep behavior disorder:** Acting out dreams as if they are real

>> **Recurrent isolated sleep paralysis:** Inability to perform voluntary movements during sleep onset or upon awakening

>> **Nightmare disorder:** Frequent, vivid, and disturbing nightmares

Other parasomnias

Other parasomnias include conditions such as

>> **Exploding head syndrome:** A loud noise or explosion sensation in the head upon waking or falling asleep

>> **Sleep-related hallucinations:** Vivid sensory phenomena that occur at the onset of sleep or upon waking

>> **Sleep-related urologic dysfunction:** Sleep *enuresis* (bed-wetting, recurrent involuntary urination during sleep occurring at least once per month for at least 3 months in individuals older than 5 years), *nocturia* (three or more nightly episodes of urination arising from sleep, followed by sleep or the intention to sleep, and lasting for at least 3 months in individuals older than 5 years), and *nocturnal urinary urge incontinence* (urinary urgency and leakage after arising from sleep, with wetness episodes occurring at least once per week for at least 3 months)

>> **Parasomnias due to a medical disorder, medication or substance, or unspecified:** For example, REM sleep behavior disorder due to the neurological disease such as Parkinson's disease, NREM parasomnias such as sleep-related eating disorder due to sleeping pills such as zolpidem (Ambien), and parasomnias that are suspected but can't be classified elsewhere with a specific diagnosis established by a physician

Recognizing parasomnia behaviors

If you notice the behaviors noted in this section in yourself or others, you may be witnessing an NREM- or REM-related parasomnia. Talk to your doctor about what's going on so that they can offer you treatment.

Sleepwalking

A person who is sleepwalking may seem totally normal in their movements, but sometimes may be slow to react to others in their environment and may bump into objects in their path. They may sleep-talk while sleepwalking, although the sleepwalker may utter only a few words, or a limited conversation may not make sense.

Sleep terrors

Even though sleep (night) terrors are most common in children, adults can experience them as well. Sleep terrors in both adults and children can potentially lead to injury due to the intense fear and physical reactions during an episode. Patients may scream, thrash, and typically don't remember the incident.

TIP

Adults who have sleep terrors may be experiencing stress, anxiety, depression, or have PTSD. Other sleep disorders that fragment sleep, such as sleep apnea or periodic limb movement disorder, can also trigger these episodes. Sleep terrors in adults can indicate an underlying problem, so if you have them, you should see a healthcare professional, especially if they happen frequently or make you or someone in your household feel unsafe.

Sleep-related eating disorder

A variant of sleepwalking, this disorder happens when you eat or drink while you're asleep, and have no memory of doing so when you wake up. For example, one of my patients used to casually drink cooking oil and converse with friends while she was asleep — and didn't remember any of it!

REM sleep behavior disorder

REM sleep behavior disorder typically manifests during REM sleep as a person physically acting out their dreams, which often involve complex scenarios. If you're the person suffering from it, you may not notice it, but if you're a bedpartner to the sufferer, you will probably be the first to notice these episodes when the individual strikes out or gets up abruptly from bed.

REM sleep behavior disorder is relatively rare, primarily affecting men in their 50s and 60s, with a prevalence of up to one percent of the general population, but the prevalence is higher in people who have associated neurological disorders. Interestingly, animals, such as cats and dogs, have shown similar behaviors while they appear to be dreaming, which can be observed on platforms such as YouTube. See Appendix B for a look at sleep study measurements that indicate REM sleep behavior disorder.

WARNING

This condition — REM sleep behavior disorder — is particularly concerning because it can precede neurological conditions such as Lewy body dementia or Parkinson's disease by several years.

Getting a diagnosis for parasomnia

You start by sharing your sleep experiences and medical history with your sleep specialist, who examines and tests you to see if your condition meets the criteria for parasomnia. In addition to the criteria for the group of NREM-related parasomnias I describe in the earlier sections, sleepwalking, sleep terrors, and sleep-related eating disorder have specific diagnostic criteria.

Sleepwalking

You experience episodes of arousal from sleep where you walk or move around (called *ambulation*) or perform other complex behaviors out of bed.

Sleep terrors

Your episodes often begin abruptly with terror, typically with an alarming vocalization, such as a frightening scream. You experience intense fear and signs of autonomic arousal, such as pupil dilation, tachycardia (increased heart rate), rapid breathing, and sweating during the episode.

Sleep-related eating disorder

You have recurrent episodes of eating after arousing during the night, during which at least one of these events happens:

You consume odd forms or combinations of food or even inedible or toxic substances.

You engage in dangerous or potentially harmful behaviors while seeking or cooking food.

You experience adverse health consequences from nocturnal eating.

You have a partial or complete lack of conscious awareness during the eating episodes, with impaired recall afterward.

Of course, the diagnosis also hinges on whether the eating disturbances are not better explained by another disorder, medication, or substance use.

REM sleep behavior disorder

You experience recurrent episodes of sleep-related vocalizations and/or complex motor behaviors, which a specialist observes during REM in an in-lab sleep study. The in-lab sleep study must demonstrate REM sleep without muscle suppression (referred to as *REM sleep without atonia*). In some cases, your specialist looks at your clinical history of acting out dreams, and presumes it occurs during REM sleep.

A sleep specialist also evaluates you for other possible parasomnias such as confusional arousals, recurrent isolated sleep paralysis, nightmare disorder, exploding head syndrome, sleep-related hallucinations, and sleep enuresis (bedwetting) based on your symptoms. And recognize that both REM sleep behavior disorder and a disorder of arousal from NREM sleep (sleepwalking or sleep terrors) may occur in an individual, in which case, that individual has what is called a *parasomnia overlap disorder*.

As always, to diagnose you with REM sleep behavior disorder, specialists must be unable to better explain your disturbances by another disease.

For example, a subtype of REM sleep behavior disorder called *status dissociates* exists, in which the affected individual (usually with an underlying neurologic or medical condition) has an extreme form of *sleep state dissociation* (where wakefulness and sleep occur simultaneously in different parts of the brain). This dissociation occurs without identifiable sleep stages, but with sleep- and dream-related behaviors that closely resemble REM sleep behavior disorder.

WARNING

You can easily confuse NREM-related parasomnias and REM-related parasomnias with other disorders that have similar symptoms. Bring with you (to your doctor's appointment) a bedpartner, family member, or friend who has witnessed the episodes or has video of the episodes to ensure a proper diagnosis by the sleep specialist.

Beyond basic sleep study diagnosis

If necessary, your sleep specialist orders you to undergo a sleep study that goes beyond the basic sleep study (which I describe in Chapter 10). It includes

>> **Expanded brain monitoring:** For this testing, a sleep specialist places extra EEG leads to check for any seizure activity, which can look a lot like NREM-related parasomnias. The EEG looks for unique signs, — such as sudden bursts of slow brain waves, EEG spikes, or brief awakenings — that might set off a parasomnia event.

>> **Safety measures:** Testing might involve extra precautions — for example, your bed might have rails — and you'll be video recorded to ensure all activity is monitored.

>> **Trigger search:** It's rare for specialists to see parasomnia happen during the study, so they focus on identifying other sleep disorders (for example, obstructive sleep apnea, or periodic limb movements during sleep) that may trigger parasomnia episodes in predisposed individuals. They also look for subtle signs, such as frequent brief awakenings during sleep and hypersynchronous delta wave activity, in which you find large, continuous delta (0.5–4 Hz) waves, that are associated with deep sleep.

Identifying associated signs and triggers (such as loud noises, lights, or internal triggers like sleep apnea or periodic limb movements) are crucial to help your doctor diagnose you. The goal of the study is to identify any underlying conditions that could precipitate these sleep disturbances for you.

Receiving treatment for parasomnia

When sleep specialists and other doctors treat you for parasomnias, there aren't many options for reducing symptoms, so they typically focus on trying to keep you and your bedpartner safe by recommending you use the following strategies:

>> **Maintain environmental safety:** Ensure the bedroom is free from harmful objects like firearms or sharp tools.

>> **Secure windows:** Lock them and place heavy drapes on them to prevent accidents, especially if your bedroom is on a higher floor.

>> **Guard stairs:** Place gates on stairway entrances to minimize the possibility of falling down stairs.

>> **Stay safe in hotels:** When traveling, choose ground-floor accommodation to minimize risks, such as falling down stairs while sleepwalking.

>> **Take preventive measures:** Try placing damp towels around the bed; the sensation of touching something cold and wet may interrupt your episode.

>> **Use door alarms:** Attach alarms to the bedroom door that can alert your bedpartner that you're up and about without waking you up (which could be dangerous in conditions like sleepwalking). The bedpartner can then gently guide you back to bed using calming words.

>> **Use soothing alarms:** Set up motion-sensitive alarms that can play the recorded soothing voice of your bedpartner or other loved one when they detect that you're out of bed.

>> **Reduce noise and light:** Use soundproof curtains and remove any bright lights from the bedroom.

>> **Treat internal triggers:** Address conditions like obstructive sleep apnea.

Regarding medication, your doctor doesn't have many options, but they may try to treat your parasomnia with

>> **Clonazepam (Klonopin):** Doctors prescribe this to increase your awakening threshold, making awakenings less likely, and reducing your deep NREM sleep. However, this medication is only about 50 percent effective and may worsen any untreated sleep apnea that you may have.

>> **Melatonin:** Doctors typically use melatonin for REM-related parasomnias, but it has shown some effectiveness for NREM-related parasomnias as well.

>> **Pramipexole (Mirapex) or transdermal rivastigmine (Exelon Patch):** Doctors may use these medications for REM-related parasomnias, but they are most commonly used for RLS.

You can find out more about sleep medications in the Appendix A.

REMEMBER

In addition to treating your symptoms, treating underlying conditions is crucial to your overall management of parasomnias.

WARNING

Treating your parasomnia isn't just a matter of your own health and safety; other people's may depend on it as well. Several known *medicolegal* (the application of medical and scientific methods as evidence) cases involve individuals who injured others while presumably sleepwalking, sometimes leading to serious harm. In the medicolegal system, such actions during sleepwalking are often classified as a *non-insane automatism*, similar to involuntary movements or actions during an epileptic seizure. If you have a sleep disorder episode that results in injury, you wouldn't necessarily be criminally liable for anything that happened during that episode, but you still wouldn't want to have that on your conscience.

Chapter **9**

Seeking Help for Your Sleep Issues

I f you already know you have sleep problems and you need help, this chapter is definitely for you. However, even if you don't think you have sleep problems, this chapter may still be for you.

You see, although sleep comprises a third of your daily life, you may not even be aware that your sleep habits are cause for concern. You may be experiencing sleep disruptions, disorders, or other problems without even knowing it, or maybe you know you don't sleep super well but that doesn't register as having sleep problems. You may think that's just how sleep is for everyone — and you're not alone. During a regular doctor's visit, patients or guardians often bring up sleep problems to their primary care physicians or pediatricians as an afterthought, versus talking about it as a primary concern.

The same goes for doctors — sleep is not always at the top of their minds to ask about. Sometimes you can go through an entire physical exam and not talk about sleep at all. But on the way out of the room, the doctor might offhandedly ask, "Oh, by the way, how's your sleep?"

In this chapter, you find out how to share your (or your child's or other dependent's) sleep concerns and other important information openly with your doctor. You also discover how to get more advanced help from a sleep clinic, and what to expect if you do find yourself in a sleep lab.

Sharing Relevant Information with Your Doctor

Sleep problems can seriously impact your daily life and long-term health, so don't hold back when talking to your doctor about them. Prioritize communicating effectively — by clearly describing lifestyle choices and habits that can affect sleep — with your healthcare provider. When you do so, you and your doctor can work together to find solutions.

TIP

Don't be afraid to advocate for yourself. Be the squeaky wheel. Speak up. You only have one life — it's up to you to live it as well as you can. Sharing as many details as possible about your sleep history and symptoms, and asking the right questions, can get you well on the road to better sleep.

Describing your sleep history and symptoms

The more information you can share with your doctor about your sleep history and symptoms, the better. Although your full history can be relevant — such as any sleep disorders you've suffered from and been treated for in the past — usually during an annual exam, your doctor will ask you to share how your sleep has been over the last year:

>> **Start with your sleep habits.** Tell your physician what your bedtime and wake times are, how long it usually takes you to fall asleep (especially if it's longer than 30 minutes), if you wake up during the night, and if so, how many times. Also let them know if you have difficulty falling back asleep and how long it takes, whether or not you have a bed partner (and if the partner disturbs your sleep), and other details about your sleep environment, such as darkness and noise levels.

>> **Tell your doctor how much stimulant or sedative substance you ingest daily.** Detail how much coffee, tea, energy drinks, chocolate, or any other

caffeine-containing you drink and eat throughout the day. Also tell them about any over-the-counter or prescription stimulants you're using (don't assume they know) — nicotine included. Note if you take anything for relaxation before sleep as well, such as alcohol, cannabis, melatonin, or herbal supplements like valerian tea.

>> **Talk about drowsiness and naps.** Your doctor should know if you experience drowsiness — while driving, at work, or other times when you should be fully awake — even after getting at least seven hours of sleep the night before. Tell them about your naps, including how often you take them, how long they are, and when you take them.

>> **Tell your doctor if you experience unusual behaviors during sleep.** Unusual behaviors can be excessive moving, hitting, or kicking (in which you hit your bed partner), periodic sleepwalking, screaming, or bedwetting. Also let them know if you have (or have been told that you have) loud disruptive snoring, stop breathing, or gasp, choke, or snort during your sleep.

>> **Share unusual behaviors, new and old.** Tell your physician if you feel a habitual urge (more than three times a week) to move your limbs that worsens at bedtime or when you are resting, but that you can temporarily relieve by moving them. Or if you suddenly feel weak during the day when you laugh, yell, get startled, or experience other strong emotions. Also, if you start going to sleep or waking up a few hours earlier or later than usual, or struggle with maintaining a consistent bedtime and morning risetime for no reason, let them know.

REMEMBER

Typically, as people age, they experience natural shifts in their sleep schedule. For example, you may find that you want to go to sleep earlier at night and get up earlier in the morning than you did when you were younger. Changes like these are usually normal, but you should still talk about them with your doctor to make sure, particularly if they interfere with your daily life.

Listing questions to ask your doctor

In addition to sharing information with your doctor, be sure to ask questions! Don't worry about looking stupid or taking up too much of the doctor's time. If there's anything at all that's bothering you or you aren't sure of regarding your sleep, ask your doctor.

TIP

Write your questions down ahead of time to make sure you cover everything in your appointment.

Some questions you might want to ask include

>> **"Given my age, are my habits like my sleep schedule within normal range?"** For example, let's say on weekdays you go to bed around eleven because you have to get up at seven every morning. But on weekends, you find that you go to sleep at two o'clock and sleep in until ten o'clock.

>> **"Am I getting enough sleep at night?"** For example, you may feel that you are not getting enough sleep, compared to your family and friends.

>> **"What are the health consequences if I have a sleep disorder?"** For example, some sleep disorders, like obstructive sleep apnea, can contribute to high blood pressure.

>> **"Can I take over-the-counter sleeping pills on nights when I'm having difficulty sleeping?"** For example, even if you don't usually like to take medications, you might have periodic sleepless nights that make you want to take a sleeping pill one or two times a week, and you want to make sure it won't harm you in the long run.

>> **"What effects does drinking alcohol at bedtime have on my sleep?"** For example, you might drink alcohol to relax or help you fall asleep at bedtime, and sometimes that can impact the quality of your sleep.

>> **"Are my symptoms like daytime sleepiness normal?"** For example, let's say you feel tired and sleepy during the day and your boss or coworkers have commented on it, or your drowsiness impacts your ability to work.

Knowing when to ask for a sleep medicine physician referral

You should ask your doctor for a referral to a sleep medicine physician if you feel that your primary care physician or pediatrician hasn't adequately addressed your (or your dependent's) sleep problem — either because you don't feel they have fully heard all of your concerns, or because their treatment isn't working for you.

If your doctor prescribes medication as a first treatment attempt, give it a fair try. If you experience side effects or the medication doesn't help, tell your doctor, and they will probably adjust the dose or try a different medication. But if you still have an issue after that and they have no other ways to treat you, ask for a referral.

TIP

If your doctor does not know how to refer you to a sleep medicine physician, there are resources that I mention later in this chapter in the section "Locating a sleep center and other online resources."

Seeing Sleep Medicine Professionals

After your doctor gives you a referral, you might want to check out the credentials and accreditations of the sleep center or sleep medicine doctor involved. You can do so easily online:

>> **To check out a sleep center's accreditation,** visit the website for the American Academy of Sleep Medicine (AASM) at www.aasm.org, which is the main sleep medicine professional organization in the United States. There you can check that the recommended sleep center is accredited by the AASM within the United States by selecting the Accreditation Verification item under the Standards & Guidelines menu, and searching for the name of your sleep center. Accredited centers have to show that they can deliver sleep evaluation and management that meet a certain standard set by the sleep medicine professional field.

>> **To confirm that the referred sleep medicine physician is board certified in sleep medicine,** you can go to the website of the American Board of Medical Specialties (ABMS) at www.abms.org, where you

1. Click on the For Patients icon and then click the Is My Doctor Board Certified button.

2. When prompted, enter your doctor's name, location, and (in the Specialty drop-down menu) click on the Sleep Medicine entry.

3. Click the Find My Doctor button.

You can alternatively go to the website for the American Board of Sleep Medicine (ABSM) at www.absm.org, where you

1. Click on the Credential Verification tab and select the Sleep Medicine menu item from the drop-down menu.

2. Click the Verify Credential button to search for your doctor's last name.

Your sleep medicine physician may have been board certified in sleep medicine through either (or both) of these organizations.

If you don't see the sleep medicine physician or center on these websites, check for a different physician or facility near your home. If the referral is listed as certified, proceed to make an appointment!

REMEMBER

If you live outside of the United States, you have other options for finding or verifying certified specialists online. You can

» **Check the website for the World Sleep Society** (WSS) at www.worldsleep society.org to find a sleep specialist. You can

1. Hover your mouse over the Programs entry in the top menu bar, then hover over the Examination option in the resulting drop-down menu.

2. After you arrive at even another menu, click on the International Sleep Specialists item in that menu.

   On the resulting page, you find a list of specialists who have earned the International Sleep Specialist designation.

» **Try the website for the European Sleep Research Society** (ESRS) at https://esrs.eu. On the site, you can

1. Hover your mouse over the Education & Events tab in the top menu bar.

2. In the resulting drop-down menu, click the Sleep Medicine Examination option under the Education category.

3. On the resulting page, scroll down to click the Certified Expert Somnologists List link under the subheading Successful Participants to search the list of certified sleep specialists.

BECOMING A SLEEP SPECIALIST

Before becoming a sleep specialist, a physician has already completed medical school — and an internship and residency — usually in internal medicine, family medicine, neurology, psychiatry, otolaryngology, head and neck surgery, pediatrics, or anesthesiology. Those who complete a residency in internal medicine may also complete additional fellowship training in pulmonary and critical care medicine. Then they go on to receive specific subspecialty training in sleep medicine during a one-year fellowship at an approved US-based institution through the Accredited Council for Graduate Medical Education (ACGME). After completing the fellowship, they can take examinations through their primary specialty board (for example, internal medicine or neurology) that is part of the American Board of Medical Specialties (ABMS) to become board-certified in sleep medicine.

Another route that a doctor can take to become a sleep specialist involves starting as a psychologist who is interested in behavioral sleep medicine. They can take a certification exam after completing behavioral sleep medicine training or a fellowship. You can find more information about becoming a sleep psychologist through the Society of Behavioral Sleep Medicine's website at www.behavioralsleep.org.

Exploring a Sleep Center

Most accredited sleep centers have two parts to them: a sleep clinic where physicians examine and evaluate patients for sleep problems, and a sleep laboratory (or sleep lab) where sleep technologists monitor patients during a sleep study.

Starting in the sleep clinic

You start the path toward your sleep diagnosis and treatment in the sleep clinic. When you walk in, you may find that the clinic feels like your primary doctor's office with a front desk, exam rooms, and medical equipment for assessments. Here you meet with your sleep medicine physician to talk about your sleep problems, medical history, and habits. The physician focuses on evaluating your sleep issues to decide on whether you need a sleep study or other treatments. They also determine what other tests, such as blood tests, you might need.

Uncovering the secrets of sleep assessment

To get the full picture of what's going on with your sleep, your sleep medicine physician uses various tools, such as questionnaires, medical history and physical exams, sleep logs and diaries, sleepiness assessments, in-lab tests, and home tests.

REMEMBER

All of these measures (which assess your situation related to sleep) can help your sleep medicine physician help you. So when taking sleep assessments, do your absolute best to be honest and participate fully and openly.

Filling out questionnaires

When you come into the sleep clinic, the front desk gives you an intake questionnaire, just like they would at any other medical practice. You write down answers to specific questions about your sleep issues, sleep habits, and overall health. It might ask about things like what time you go to bed, whether you snore or exhibit unusual movements or behaviors as reported by your bed partner, or if you feel tired or sleepy during the day.

You also typically find a section that includes the *Epworth Sleepiness Scale,* a set of questions that asks you to rate your tendency to doze during eight different real-life scenarios on a scale of zero to three. Your answers help guide your provider to pinpoint your level of daytime sleepiness and what type of sleep disorders you might have.

Fleshing out sleep history and physical condition

The sleep medicine physician takes a full medical history that focuses on your sleep and related health. In addition to the general information you share with your primary care doctor about your sleep, your sleep medicine physician may want information about various symptoms you experience — from waking up with a dry mouth to having difficulty falling or staying asleep. If you would like the full details on these symptoms and many others you can expect your physician to explore further, turn to Chapters 7 and 8.

To accompany the assessment, your physician conducts a standard physical exam to check your heart rate, listen to your breathing, and examine your throat and mouth for signs of sleep-related issues such as sleep apnea.

REMEMBER

A physician may also look for other physical factors that could affect your sleep, such as obesity, nasal congestion, and neurological signs. For example, tremors, gait instability, or rigidity are symptoms of Parkinson's disease which can significantly affect your sleep because it is associated with certain sleep disorders such as REM sleep behavior disorder.

Keeping sleep logs or diaries

Before your sleep study, your doctor might ask you to keep a sleep log (also called a diary) to track your sleep habits on a nightly basis over a course of time (up to two weeks) leading up to your lab visit. Typically, they want you to track

>> The times you go to bed and wake up

>> How long it takes you to fall asleep

>> How many times you think that you woke up during the night

>> How many total minutes or hours you spent awake during the time that you were in bed

>> How alert you feel during the daytime on a rating scale

>> Anything unusual that happened during the day or night that might have affected your alertness or sleep

You bring your sleep log or diary with you to your appointment at the sleep clinic or lab, and your sleep medicine physician later reviews it to help get a complete picture of your sleep patterns and any sleep-related issues you experience. You can find a downloadable template of a sleep diary on the NIH (National Heart, Lung and Blood Institute) website at www.nhlbi.nih.gov/resources/sleep-diary. It looks something like the depiction in Figure 9-1, which shows a sample entry.

Sleep Diary

	June 13				
Today's date:	June 13				
Number of caffeinated drinks (coffee, tea, cola) and time when I had them today:	1 drink, 8 p.m.				
Number of alcoholic drinks (beer, wine, liquor) and time when I had them today:	2 drinks, 9 p.m.				
Naptimes and lengths today:	3:30 p.m., 45 minutes				
Exercise times and lengths today:	None				
How sleepy did I feel during the day today? 1—So sleepy I had to struggle to stay awake during much of the day 2—Somewhat tired 3—Fairly alert 4—Alert	1				
Today's date:	June 14				
• Time I went to bed last night:	11 p.m.				
• Time I got out of bed this morning:	7 a.m.				
• Hours spent in bed last night:	8				
Number of awakenings and total time awake last night:	5 times, 2 hours				
How long I took to fall asleep last night:	30 minutes				
Medicines taken last night:	None				
How alert did I feel when I got up this morning? 1—Alert 2—Alert but a little tired 3—Sleepy	2				

Fill out before going to bed (first section)
Fill out in the morning (second section)

FIGURE 9-1: A sleep diary template with sample entry.

REMEMBER

Do your best to maintain a regular sleep-wake schedule for the two weeks leading up to the sleep study appointment, but always be honest in your sleep log/diary. Don't worry that your entries in the sleep log/diary might seem wrong; the goal is to record the timing and regularity of your sleep schedule.

Getting cozy in the sleep lab

After consulting with your sleep medicine physician in the clinic, you will most likely find that the physician orders a sleep study for you to complete on a future visit. For that study, you go to the sleep lab, which could be part of the sleep clinic, part of a hospital or university medical center, or a freestanding independent facility nearby.

The lab is set up like a bedroom or hotel room, equipped with comfortable beds, dim lighting, and sometimes amenities like a television and desk to simulate a home-like environment. During the study, you spend the night, and the lab personnel monitor your sleep to learn more about the quantity and quality of your sleep. (You sometimes stay in the lab part or all of the next day to monitor your alertness and sleepiness levels if so ordered by your sleep medicine physician; see the section "Assessing Objective Sleep and Sleepiness" later in the chapter.)

Sleep lab personnel attach sensors and recording equipment to your face, head, and body to record various physiological parameters such as

>> Brain waves

>> Heart rate

>> Oxygen levels

>> Breathing patterns

>> Movements while you sleep

Sleep technologists oversee these studies from a separate control room, monitoring the data in real time.

When your physician orders a sleep study, you should bring with you (to the sleep lab) an overnight bag that contains items specific to your treatment and also many of the items that you may normally pack for an overnight trip, including

>> Paperwork related to the study, including sleep logs (find more on that in the section "Keeping sleep logs or diaries" earlier in this chapter)

>> ID and insurance card

>> Any prescription medication (*Note:* Lab personnel may ask you to take some of your medications before you arrive at the lab, as long as they are not sedating medications that could make you sleepy while driving.)

>> Modest and comfortable pajamas

>> Clothes for the next day

>> Snacks

>> Reading material, phone, or computer to pass the time when awake

>> Personal hygiene items

WARNING

When you come to the sleep lab for a study, do not bring valuables, pets (aside from a service animal, but check with the sleep laboratory ahead of your visit), or guests (aside from a pre-approved caregiver if needed). Also, you might want to arrange for someone to pick you up in the morning (for example, a family member or rideshare service) because you might be too sleepy to drive.

Knowing who's who in the sleep center

In addition to your sleep medicine physician, many other professionals work in or with a sleep center, either in the sleep clinic or lab:

>> **CCSH: Certified Clinical Sleep Health educators** work directly with patients, families, and providers to coordinate and manage patient care. They also assist in educating the patients regarding their condition and care management.

>> **RPSGT/RST: Registered Polysomnographic Technologists (RPSGTs) and Registered Sleep Technologists** (RSTs) receive training in sleep disorder evaluation and are responsible for managing patients during sleep studies as well as scoring the sleep studies. The training requirements are similar for both RPSGTs and RSTs.

>> **CRT/RRT: Respiratory Therapists** come in three types, but you usually see only two types in the sleep lab: Certified Respiratory Therapists (CRTs) and Registered Respiratory Therapists (RRTs). They receive training in critical care and cardiopulmonary medicine, and — similar to RPSGTs/RSTs — are responsible for managing patients during sleep studies as well as scoring the sleep studies. RRTs generally practice more independently and receive more respiratory training than CRTs.

TIP

Usually, you find one technologist (either RPSGT/RST or CRT/RRT) for every two patients in a sleep lab unless a patient has very complex medical issues. In that case, the ratio will be one to one.

Meeting the professionals in sequence

Most likely, you meet the sleep center professionals in the order presented in Table 9-1 as you go through the diagnostic and study processes.

Sleep lab personnel work 24/7, meaning that they work in multiple shifts. So when you check into the sleep laboratory (which is most likely in the evening), the technologist with you at night may not be the same technologist you see in the morning.

TABLE 9-1   ## Sleep Center Professionals

Interaction Sequence	Who They Are	What They Do
1	Front desk staff: administrative employees and medical assistants	Set up appointments, handle insurance, keep patient records, and facilitate information flow between all parties. They get you checked in and answer any immediate questions you have.
2	Sleep medicine physician: fully credentialed doctor (often a pulmonologist, psychiatrist, internist, family practitioner, otolaryngologist, pediatrician, or neurologist) with additional credentials in sleep medicine	Consult with you, order sleep studies, review test results, issue diagnoses, and recommend treatments, including follow-up visits. Allied health professionals, including nurse practitioners and physician assistants, or sleep medicine trainees (fellows and residents) may work with the physician.
3	Behavioral sleep medicine psychologist	Treats you with cognitive behavioral therapy (CBT-1) via a referral from a sleep medicine physician if you have insomnia.
4	Sleep technologist (RST, RPSGT) and/or respiratory therapist (CRT, RRT)	Run the sleep studies, including Applying sensors and recording instruments on your body that communicate with lab equipment Dispensing necessary questionnaires to you before bedtime and in the morning Accommodating patient requests, such as assistance to and from the bathroom at night
5	Scoring technologist (RST, RPGST, CRT, RRT, CCSH)	Score or code all of the data from the sleep study (whether onsite or remote) so that your sleep medicine physician can review and interpret the results and give you a diagnosis and full treatment plan.
6	Sleep health educator (RST, RPSGT, CRT, RRT, CCSH)	Provide additional coaching following diagnosis to make sure you understand your sleep disorder by Explaining your disorder, how newly prescribed devices (such as PAP) work, and how to properly use the equipment Following up with you after you receive the equipment to address usage issues
7	Durable medical equipment (DME) provider or supplier (RST, RPSGT, CRT, RRT, CCSH)	Deliver your PAP therapy devices and oxygen delivery systems to your home, and give you support throughout your treatment as your needs and PAP technologies change. Although DMEs are typically part of a healthcare company (local or national) and usually work outside of the sleep lab, an individual representative may be present in the lab to help explain and streamline the process.

WARNING

Not all sleep centers have registered nurses (RNs) on staff. If you have home healthcare or other regular services with a nursing component, ask during sleep clinic or sleep study scheduling whether you must bring your nurse or caregiver with you.

Spending the night in a sleep lab

Your time in the sleep lab will probably go something like this:

1. **Check in with the front desk and fill out paperwork.**

Your assigned sleep technologist meets with you to go over the plan for the evening and answer questions. They explain how they monitor and videotape you during your stay to record any unusual movements while you're asleep.

2. **Get settled into your assigned bedroom.**

The sleep technologist helps you settle in, shows you where to put your personal items, and connects you to equipment by applying sensors and other recording instruments to your face, head, and body. They typically request that you complete a bedtime questionnaire asking about any daytime activities, recent illnesses, medications, or other issues that might affect your sleep during the study.

3. **Go to sleep (usually at or close to your regular bedtime).**

Sleep lab personnel show you how to reach out to the technologists, who are typically in an adjoining room. If you need assistance during the night, you can usually press a bedside button, like the ones used in a hospital.

4. **Wake up at the urging of the sleep technologist(s), typically close to your usual awakening time.**

At that time, you complete a morning questionnaire asking about your night's sleep. Additionally, the technologist removes the sensors and recording instruments from you. Before you leave the lab, the technologist also informs you when you can expect to receive the sleep study results.

Undergoing daytime testing in a sleep lab

In addition to the nighttime data that technologists collect, your technologist may run one or both of two primary in-laboratory tests during the day as well:

>> **The Multiple Sleep Latency Test (MSLT),** which is a series of up to five scheduled naps designed to evaluate your propensity to fall asleep, and the MSLT follows the overnight sleep study. These 20-minute naps occur at two-hour intervals throughout the day. The electrodes from your overnight study may still be attached, with some adjustments made, as necessary.

In a controlled, dark environment, the technician instructs you to lie quietly in a comfortable position with your eyes closed and attempt to sleep. The MSLT aids in diagnosing conditions such as narcolepsy and idiopathic hypersomnia (see more about these disorders in Chapter 7). If you need to take this test, it generally happens immediately following your night in the lab.

>> **The Maintenance of Wakefulness Test (MWT),** which measures your ability to stay awake. This test includes four 40-minute trials, each spaced two hours apart, in which you are seated in a semi-darkened room. This setting simulates real-life situations (like driving) that require you to remain alert. The MWT may follow the overnight sleep study and may be required for professional drivers or pilots to ensure safety in a job situation. Characteristics of MWT testing include

- *Careful supervision of your actions:* If you go through the MWT test, expect your technician to check on you regularly to make sure that you're not artificially enhancing your wakefulness. For example, if you say during one of your breaks, "Oh, I'm going to leave the lab for a moment," you may be escorted, just to make sure that you're not taking a stimulant, or getting your blood pumping by running around the block or something.

- *Explicit instructions for your activity:* For the MWT, the technologist instructs you to stay in a sitting position and remain awake for as long as possible, but not to resort to any movements or behaviors specifically to stay awake.

If you need the MWT test, you may not necessarily have to spend the night in the sleep lab the night beforehand. Your sleep medicine physician decides and discusses this with you ahead of time so you can properly prepare for this test.

REMEMBER

To prepare for these daytime tests, maintain a consistent sleep schedule and avoid medications or substances that could affect sleepiness (whether they are stimulants or sedatives) for two weeks prior to the study. And don't try to fool anyone — the sleep lab staff runs a urine toxicology screen to ensure that you have nothing in your system to interfere with the testing.

If you're unwell with a cold (or other sickness) or if you otherwise experience a change in your condition, inform the sleep medicine physician who ordered the test. The physician will then decide whether you should proceed with the test or reschedule it.

Understanding these procedures and adhering to the preparation guidelines will help ensure the accuracy of your sleep study results.

In some instances, your technologist may cancel your daytime tests. One of the more common reasons for cancellation occurs when you don't have six or more hours of objective sleep the night before and are more sleepy than usual. Another reason may be that you have a strong reason for being sleepy and the technician witnesses this during your nighttime testing. For example, you may exhibit obstructive sleep apnea, or frequent periodic limb movements that cause brief awakenings during sleep.

Assessing Sleep and Sleepiness Objectively

Objective assessments of sleep and wakefulness rely on measuring and recording actual sleep or body activity as a measure of sleep and wakefulness (rather than subjective reporting about your sleep situation) and are essential in unraveling the complexities of sleep health and related disorders. Specialists use a variety of instruments to measure your body's activity. They may give you an *actigraph* to wear at home, typically on your wrist, which functions as a movement detector. This device helps your doctor estimate your sleep and wake patterns, and you might need to wear it for a few weeks before getting a sleep study. For a deeper understanding of how this technology works, flip to Chapter 10.

Conducting home sleep tests

Your doctor may also recommend a home sleep test to objectively assess your breathing during sleep. I cover more about how home sleep tests work in Chapter 9, but basically, you use a limited device to assess specific sleep-related breathing disorders such as obstructive sleep apnea. The sleep lab gives you the device to bring home and wear for one night — sometimes two — and then you bring it back to the lab, where the staff can download and review the data.

In some cases, you may not need to visit the sleep lab to pick up and return equipment for a home sleep test, because the lab can mail a disposable home sleep test to you. Through your Wi-Fi connection, these tests can upload the data gathered to the cloud for the lab to access. This practice became popular during the COVID-19 pandemic of 2020.

Blood tests and cerebrospinal fluid (CSF) tests

Although the MSLT (see its description in section "Undergoing daytime testing in a sleep lab" earlier in the chapter) is really the gold standard for diagnosing narcolepsy, your doctor may conduct blood or cerebrospinal fluid (CSF) tests if they need extra information to assess whether you might have narcolepsy.

>> **For a blood test,** technicians draw blood from one of your arm veins, which only takes a few minutes. Then your sample goes to the lab for a human leukocyte antigen (HLA) profile, where the lab techs check to find out whether you have specific genetic markers for narcolepsy. Not all genetic markers and tests are created equal, though. Some are excellent for detecting narcolepsy type 1, but not as good for narcolepsy type 2. So if your doctor suspects you may have narcolepsy, they might order this blood test, but not always.

>> **For a cerebral lumbar puncture (spinal tap),** your doctor may opt for this procedure, because it provides better and stronger clarity for diagnosing narcolepsy. It measures the level of hypocretin-1 (also known as orexin-A) in your cerebrospinal fluid. *Hypocretin-1* is a *neuropeptide* (a chemical messenger) involved in the sleep/wake cycle in humans. If you have low levels (at or below 110 picograms per milliliter), that situation could indicate that you have narcolepsy type 1. However, it isn't as reliable for narcolepsy type 2, so your doctor may only do the CSF test if your MSLT results and clinical symptoms are unclear.

WARNING

Very few labs are able to process CSF samples for hypocretin-1/orexin-A, and the wait time for results might be weeks to months, even in top labs like Stanford.

Your doctor may also order:

>> **Thyroid function tests.** If your thyroid levels are low (*hypothyroidism*), this condition may lead to sleepiness.

>> **Ferritin (iron) tests.** If you have iron deficiency, anemia, and low ferritin, that situation can be associated with restless legs syndrome (RLS).

Locating a sleep center and other online resources

The American Academy of Sleep Medicine (AASM) has online educational resources you can check out at `https://sleepeducation.org`. It is the best place to go if you want to learn more about sleep disorders and how to locate sleep centers accredited by the AASM. You can also check the Patient Information section of their main website at https://aasm.org. Click the Patients tab in the top menu of the site to reach the patient information.

Additionally, the National Sleep Foundation also has a website at www.thensf.org whose main purpose is patient education. They have information about sleep health, including how to improve your sleep and data from their annual Sleep in America Polls (that you can find under the Research menu option), which assesses the sleep health of the United States population.

Many individual sleep centers and sleep disorders also have their own websites that provide education and patient support. And some patient education and support organizations exist for specific sleep disorders, such as the Restless Legs Syndrome Foundation, which you can find at www.rls.org.

4

Assessing Sleep Technology

Chapter **10**

Discovering Technology in the Sleep Clinic and Laboratory

Technology plays a significant role in the world of sleep medicine. Sleep specialists and technologists use multiple devices and tools to accurately monitor and analyze your sleep patterns and other bodily functions that change during sleep so they can give you the most accurate diagnosis possible.

In this chapter, I guide you through how various diagnostic equipment works, including the *polysomnography* machines, which capture your brain waves, eye movements, muscle activity, and other measures while you sleep. I also cover the simpler actigraphy devices that track your overall sleep-wake cycles. Getting to know the importance of each piece of equipment in diagnosing and managing sleep disorders helps you understand and prepare for what happens during a sleep study.

Innovations like portable monitoring devices allow you to receive home sleep testing, which can be a convenient option for helping your sleep specialist diagnose *obstructive sleep apnea* and other sleep-related breathing conditions (refer to Chapter 8 for more information).

Measuring Sleep and Other Parameters with Polysomnography

Polysomnography (PSG) is the technology your sleep specialist uses during a day-time or nighttime in-laboratory sleep study to measure the way your body functions during sleep. They can use PSGs to

>> **Identify sleep disorders** through a *diagnostic PSG/sleep study*, which enables the sleep specialist to identify and subsequently diagnose sleep disorders by analyzing the data obtained through this study.

>> **Treat obstructive, central, or mixed sleep apnea** by involving mechanisms such as continuous positive airway pressure (CPAP), bilevel positive airway pressure (BPAP), adaptive servo ventilation (ASV), or average volume-assured pressure support (AVAPS).

REMEMBER

Sleep specialists also call this treatment portion of a PSG a *titration PSG/sleep study* or a *split-night PSG/sleep study* — a study in which the first part of the test is a diagnostic PSG, and the second part is a titration of pressure for the treatment segment. A split-night PSG/sleep study can also use an oral appliance such as a *mandibular advancement device* (which is a mouthguard/retainer that clips on to the teeth before sleep and positions the lower jaw forward to open the airway) instead of CPAP, BPAP, ASV, or AVAPS in the second part of the study.

You can see examples of a CPAP and an oral appliance in Chapter 8. The purpose of these titration studies is usually to adjust the settings and pressures of these devices during the study in order to optimize how well they treat your sleep-related breathing disorder.

In addition to measuring your actual sleep, sleep specialists perform a nighttime PSG to look at breathing and any unusual behavior during sleep. Figure 10-1 shows the setup of a typical room where a sleep-study patient would spend the night in a sleep clinic.

Your specialist may also order a *multiple sleep latency test* (MSLT) or *maintenance of wakefulness test* (MWT), which, when combined with the data from the nighttime PSG, will help the specialist diagnose your sleep disorder(s). For the MSLT or MWT, specialists primarily rely on EEG, EOG, EMG, and heart rate measurements. To read about the MSLT and MWT in detail, turn to Chapter 9.

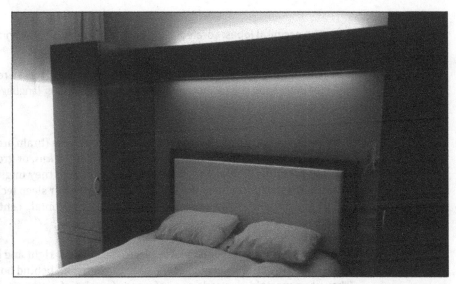

FIGURE 10-1:
Sleeping
arrangements in
a clinic where a
sleep study
patient spends
the night.

Photo courtesy of Clete A. Kushida

REMEMBER

Specialists do not analyze your breathing during (MSLT and MWT) daytime tests because they use these tests to diagnose sleep problems or disorders other than sleep-related breathing disorders. The main questions that these daytime tests answer are

>> **For MSLT:** How quickly do you fall asleep?

>> **For MWT:** How long can you stay awake?

Electroencephalography (EEG)

To perform *electroencephalography* (one component of the PSG testing), technologists place electrodes at measured distances on the scalp overlying certain brain regions called *lobes*. These include

>> **The frontal lobes:** This region is in charge of aspects of personality, decision-making, movement, attention, and memory, as well as motor tasks, judgment, abstract thinking, creativity, and social appropriateness.

>> **Parietal lobes:** Located in the middle of your brain, they help you identify objects and process sensory information, language, and spatial relations.

>> **The occipital lobes:** Located in the back of the brain, they're primarily responsible for vision, color properties, and visual memory.

>> **The temporal lobes:** Located on the side of your brain, they're responsible for processing auditory information, memory, emotions, language, and visual processing.

Technologists also place electrodes on the *prefrontal area* (brain area at the front of the frontal lobe) and the *central area* (above the *central sulcus*, or groove in the brain that separates the frontal and parietal lobes). Although they might use electrodes at any of the noted locations, for most sleep studies, your sleep technologist places electrodes on your scalp over your left and right frontal, central, and occipital areas.

Additionally, the technologist places electrodes on your right and left *mastoid processes* (the bony bumps located at the base of your skull behind both of your ears). They use a mastoid electrode as a reference (a point of comparison for measuring the electrical activity recorded by another active electrode) for the electrical signals from the brain. Typically technologists reference the right frontal, central, and occipital electrodes to the left mastoid electrode, and vice versa, so that they can monitor and record the EEG from both sides of your brain during the sleep study. Figure 10-2 shows recommended locations for placement of electrodes on the scalp during a sleep study.

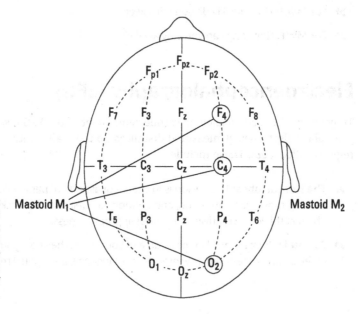

FIGURE 10-2: Recommended EEG derivations for recording EEG during a PSG by the American Academy of Sleep Medicine.

The EEG electrodes record your brain waves as you sleep. Your specialist analyzes the tracing of these waves in 30-second intervals called *epochs*. They look for how often (*frequency*) and how high (*amplitude*) these waves appear in each 30-second epoch. Sleep specialists measure the frequency in Hertz (Hz, how many cycles per second) and categorize them into different frequency bands:

>> **Delta waves (0.5 to 4 Hz):** These are the slowest waves, typically associated with stage NREM (non-REM) N3 sleep (turn to Chapter 2 to read more about the different stages of sleep).

>> **Theta waves (4 to 8 Hz):** These waves usually show up in lighter stages of sleep and also during periods of drowsiness.

>> **Alpha waves (8 to 13 Hz):** Alpha waves appear in states of wakefulness and alertness, but they can also be present in REM sleep (but usually at a slower frequency than waking alpha waves).

>> **Beta waves (13 to 30 Hz):** Beta waves show during active, alert states of consciousness.

By examining these waves, specialists can distinguish between wakefulness and sleep EEG wave patterns. Reviewing the waveform data along with the eye and chin movements (which I discuss in the following sections "Electrooculography (EOG)" and "Electromyography (EMG)") helps determine sleep versus wake times and detect various stages of sleep, as well as helping sleep specialists understand how well you're sleeping and identify any issues that might be affecting your sleep quality.

Electrooculography (EOG)

To perform electrooculography (EOG) — another piece of the PSG measurements — sleep technologist places electrodes on the *outer (lateral) canthus* of each eye, which is the outer corner of the eye where the upper and lower eyelids meet. The electrodes used in EOG include

>> One electrode 1 centimeter below and 1 centimeter lateral to the left outer canthus

>> One electrode 1 centimeter above and 1 centimeter lateral to the right outer canthus

>> Reference mastoid electrodes (as used for the EEG described in the previous section) which reference the right outer canthus electrodes to the left mastoid electrode, and vice versa

REM SLEEP AND EYE MOVEMENTS

Because the cornea at the front of the eye is electrically positive with respect to the retina at the back of the eye (which is electrically negative), when an individual looks to the right, the right outer canthus electrode will register a positive electrical signal, and the left outer canthus electrode will register a negative electrical signal (for more information about measuring eye movements, turn to Chapter 2). The EOG electrical signals on the PSG are reflective of the specific placement of the electrodes on the outer canthi of both eyes and the positive and negative polarity of the eyes. This allows the technologist and sleep specialist to tell the directionality of the eye movements (i.e., left, right, up, and down).

When both eyes move simultaneously in the same direction (as they normally do during wakefulness and sleep), these are called *in-phase* eye movements. However, when recording eye movements with EOG, out-of-phase electrical signals are seen on the EOG due to the different electrical potentials generated by each eye. During REM sleep, the EOG displays clusters of rapid eye movements that may correspond to dream content (for example, if — during a dream — the individual is looking for an airplane in the sky, the eye movements on the EOG will reflect this event).

EOG allows your sleep specialist to monitor the eye movements that occur when you're alert and looking around, the slow and rolling eye movements when you're falling asleep, and the rapid eye movements that are characteristic during dreaming in REM sleep.

Electromyography (EMG)

A sleep technologist uses electromyography (EMG) to measure muscle activity in various parts of your body during a PSG/sleep study. They attach electrodes to measure this muscle activity, including one or more of these:

>> **Chin muscle activity.** Specialists measure this activity by placing electrodes at various locations on your mandible (jawbone):

- *Mental:* In the midline of the chin, 1 centimeter above the mandible's *inferior edge* (the bottom of the jawbone)

- *Submental left:* 2 centimeters below the mandible's inferior edge, 2 centimeters to the left of the midline

- *Submental right:* 2 centimeters below the mandible's inferior edge, 2 centimeters to the right of the midline

>> **Jaw muscle activity.** If your sleep specialist suspects you have *bruxism* (teeth grinding), they can track your jaw muscle activity by placing EMG electrodes on your *masseters* (the muscles in your cheeks that close your jaw).

>> **Neck muscle activity.** Your specialist may place EMG electrodes on specific locations such as the back of your neck to measure muscle activity if your specialist suspects rhythmic movements during sleep.

>> **Leg and arm movements.** Your sleep specialist may also measure activity in your legs by placing EMG electrodes on your left and right *anterior tibialis muscles* (the long, thick, fleshy muscles in the front of your shin bone that run from below your knee to the top of your foot). And sometimes, your sleep specialist may measure your arm movements by placing EMG electrodes on your left and right flexor *digitorum superficialis* (the large forearm muscle that bends the fingers).

Other measures involved in PSG

Sleep specialists also measure the activity related to your heart and respiration during a PSG/sleep study. Again, they attach devices to your body when they measure

>> **Your heart's activity,** specifically, your cardiac rhythm or cardiac rate. They measure this by placing two electrodes called the *single modified ECG lead II* on the torso.

>> **Your airflow, respiratory effort, and blood oxygenation.** To measure your breathing by recording airflow from your nose to mouth, they place a *nasal pressure transducer* (a tube with prongs that sits under your nose and partially into your nostrils) to measure pressure variability associated with breathing and/or *nasal thermal airflow sensors* (temperature-sensitive wires that fit partially into your nose and in front of the mouth) to measure airflow from your nose and mouth).

To record your breathing effort measurements, they place bands or belts on your chest and abdomen. These bands respond to variations in resistance with changes in body circumference, allowing your specialist to measure how hard your chest and abdomen work during breathing.

They measure your oxygenation by using *a pulse oximeter*, which is basically an electronic finger probe that they clip to the outside of your finger. This probe has a light source that passes light through the finger, and by analyzing this transmitted light the device is able to determine the percentage of oxygen in the blood.

Pulse oximeters can give variations on their readings depending on the skin color of the patient, so talk to your doctor about how they plan to address that issue if you have concerns.

Don't wear fingernail polish or any cosmetic coverings on your finger, as those items may interfere with the oximeter reading.

Measurements specific to diagnosing apnea

In some cases, your specialist might use *esophageal manometry*, in which they insert a small *cannula* (a thin tube) into your nose. They position the cannula's tip in your esophagus. This helps them assess how hard you work to breathe by detecting breathing-related pressure variation in your chest that's transmitted into the esophagus. A targeted measurement like this can help your specialist determine which type of apnea you may have. For example, if they detect pauses in your diaphragm activity, you may have central apneas versus obstructive apneas.

Specialists also sometimes use *transcutaneous* or *end-tidal carbon dioxide monitoring* to detect conditions such as *obesity hypoventilation syndrome*, a type of abnormal breathing during sleep that affects those who are overweight. If patients have this breathing condition, they are unable to breathe deeply or rapidly, resulting in low oxygen levels and high carbon dioxide levels in the blood.

For the transcutaneous carbon dioxide sensor, the specialist typically places an electrode on the skin of your cheek, and for the end-tidal carbon dioxide sensor they typically put small tubes under your nose. These sensors and tubes connect to equipment that monitors your carbon dioxide levels.

If your child is the one receiving these tests, keep in mind that the assessment methods for children and adults differ mainly in the scoring of signals rather than the recording instrumentation the specialists use.

How all these measurements affect each other

A computer picks up all of the signals from all types of PSG, and then the sleep technologists review these signals. First, they score your sleep in 30-second segments, called *epochs* (see the section "Electroencephalography (EEG)" earlier in the chapter). They assign each epoch a sleep stage, and within the epoch, they also identify abnormal breathing events, cardiac arrhythmias, and unusual movements during sleep.

When you move or change body positions during sleep, a lot of *artifacts* — which are noises or signals that can disturb your EEG, EOG, EMG, or ECG recordings — can occur. These may include

>> **Sixty-cycle interference,** which is a common artifact that comes from space heaters or other electronic equipment.

>> **Artifacts from respiratory or cardiac activity,** which can happen when your electrodes become partially dislodged and the equipment picks up the artifacts. For example, in the EEG, specialists might see cardiac signals or fluctuations due to respiratory effort.

A typical sleep lab minimizes sixty-cycle interference and checks for other artifacts due to movement by using filtering (which in the early days of PSG were manual filters, but now are digital filters) to screen out some of this interference.

In addition to the signals discussed for polysomnography, sleep specialists also monitor your body position. Body position is important, especially in sleep-disordered breathing conditions, because symptoms can worsen when you're lying on your back. They also record snoring sounds using microphones or electrodes placed above the trachea and sometimes use intercostal EMG electrodes to help them analyze your breathing. And your sleep study may also involve videotaping you during the night to record any unusual movements or behaviors that you demonstrate. Figure 10-3 shows a sleep clinic control room and the equipment required to keep track of all the various aspects of sleep that a sleep study monitors.

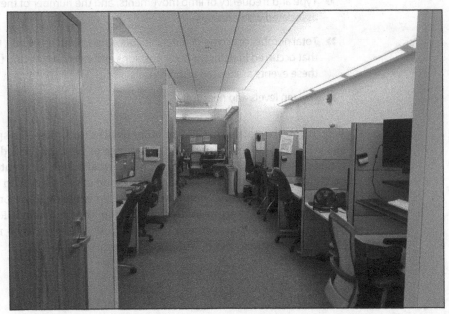

FIGURE 10-3:
The sleep clinic control room.

Photo courtesy of Clete A. Kushida

Getting your PSG sleep study results

After the sleep study, you receive your results, sleep disorder diagnosis, and next steps, either via a message from the lab or at an in-person visit. The results of the sleep studies are quite comprehensive and include these data:

>> Lights off (bedtime) and lights on (awakening time)

>> Time in bed (time span from lights off to lights on)

>> Total sleep time (the time that you're actually asleep)

>> Wake after sleep onset (amount of wake time during the study, including the number of *arousals* (brief awakenings)) from the time first asleep to lights on

>> Sleep efficiency, which is the percentage calculated by dividing the time spent asleep by the time in bed and multiplying by 100 (for example, 7 hours asleep divided by a time in bed of 8 hours, and then multiplied by 100, results in a sleep efficiency of 87.5 percent)

>> Time in different sleep stages, percentages of these sleep stages over total sleep time, and how long it took you to enter into the stages of sleep (sleep latency and REM sleep latency)

>> Time you spent in different body positions

>> Type and frequency of limb movements, and the number of these events associated with arousals

>> Total number and type of different abnormal breathing events, the number that occurred in different body positions and sleep stages, and the number of these events associated with arousals

>> Oxygen levels and heart rate

Note: If you are started on CPAP or other devices (or if the sleep specialist wants to test whether you are on the optimal settings of CPAP or these devices), the specialist obtains the type and number of abnormal breathing events that occur with each change in pressure as well as the duration of sleep stages in which the events occur. Assessing whether you have REM sleep while on CPAP or other devices is particularly important; in this situation, you should obtain a *REM sleep rebound* (more REM sleep than without these devices) and experience minimized or no abnormal breathing events with these devices.

Finding Out About Home Sleep Tests

An alternative to the in-laboratory sleep study (see the section "Measuring Sleep and Other Parameters with Polysomnography" earlier in the chapter) is *home sleep tests* (HSTs). Although HSTs — also called *home sleep apnea tests (HSATs), portable monitoring (PM)*, or *out-of-center sleep tests (OCSTs)* — may have the word *sleep* in their name, it's a bit of a misnomer because many of the devices don't detect or measure sleep; they may simply estimate it.

The equipment does the estimating, for example, by using measures such as changes in heartrate that differ between wakefulness and sleep or recording activity and *lack of activity*, which it calls *sleep*. However, in the latter example, this lack of activity may result from the patient lying quietly in bed, but the equipment has no way to be sure.

HST helps your specialist diagnose obstructive sleep apnea (OSA), a condition where you temporarily stop breathing while you're sleeping (to read more on that, turn to Chapter 8). To perform HST, you set up a portable device yourself at home before going to sleep based on instructions, handouts, or videos provided to you by your sleep specialist.

Figure 10-4 shows a WatchPAT ONE home testing device as depicted on the Zoll Itamar website at (www.itamar-medical.com/professionals/disposable-hsawatchpat-one). A device like this uses technology named *peripheral arterial tonometry* (PAT, which measures arterial blood volume in the peripheral vascular bed in the fingertip that changes with the pulse) and other equipment which directly or indirectly measures your airflow, breathing effort, blood oxygen levels, heart rate, and body position to assess OSA.

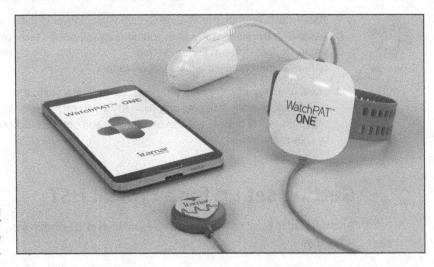

FIGURE 10-4: WatchPAT ONE home testing device.

While HST provides fewer comprehensive data than full polysomnography in a sleep lab, it offers the benefits of being less cumbersome for the patient and often more affordable. Home testing works best if you have clear signs of sleep apnea and no other serious medical conditions or suspected sleep disorders. HST has become increasingly popular because it allows you to sleep in your familiar surroundings, making the testing process more comfortable and potentially more reflective of your normal sleep behavior.

Examining the levels of HST devices

The process begins with you receiving a portable device, either in person at the lab or through a home delivery. These portable devices belong to one of four classifications, called levels or types. The different levels of devices used for home sleep testing are

>> **Level I or Type I:** Devices at this level typically include 14 or more electrodes or sensors such as EEG, EOG, EMG, ECG, airflow, effort, and oximetry. Level I is the highest level and is what technologists use in the sleep center.

>> **Level II or Type II:** Devices at this level are similar to Level I devices but they are called *unattended* (technologists don't attend them, and you can use them in the home environment). You find about a dozen of these devices on the market.

>> **Level III or Type III:** The most common portable devices for home use, this level typically comes with four to six electrodes or sensors that measure airflow, respiratory effort, oximetry, and ECG/heart rate. These devices are unattended, so technologists don't monitor this device in real time; they review the data later. Level III devices for FDA approval must be reliable and accurate in detecting sleep disorders, particularly sleep-related breathing disorders.

These most common portable devices offer you convenient at-home use and a cost-effective sleep study. Plus, you don't always need a technologist to hook up the devices. You can find more than 30 models that are currently commercially available and used by sleep laboratories.

>> **Level IV or Type IV:** These unattended devices have one to three electrodes or sensors, typically including only oximetry, heart rate, and/or airflow. Studies that use Level IV devices are also unattended and not as comprehensive as studies that use Level III.

Getting set up for a typical HST

Your specialist prescribes a commonly used Level III device for your home sleep study if you

>> **Have a high probability of having a sleep-related breathing disorder** such as moderate to severe obstructive sleep apnea.

>> **Don't need a technologist-attended, in-laboratory sleep study** due to the absence of serious *comorbidities* (simultaneously existing disease or medical conditions) such as heart failure or stroke.

>> **Are not suspected of having other sleep disorders,** such as *parasomnias* (unusual behaviors during sleep) or *periodic limb movement disorder* (frequent repetitive limb movements during sleep). Your specialist can detect these other disorders by Level I or II studies but not by Level III or IV studies.

Your sleep specialists can study you from your home, often after you come in for a 30-minute (or longer) hookup (otherwise known as *electrode and sensor application*) session, during which you

>> **Receive the device** and an explanation of what the device does

>> **Get instruction on** how to apply the device

>> **Find out what to do** with the device after the test is complete

Sometimes the technologist might even put on some of the electrodes or sensors for you, if they need to go in an area where they're difficult to apply, such as the chest. However, some of the devices can be less obtrusive, such as a ring you wear on your finger. Typically, you wear some of these devices for just one night, but some can collect your data over the course of more than one night.

Many different Level III devices exist, and sometimes — instead of picking up the device from the lab — the lab can ship it to you with instructions and sometimes a link to instructional videos.

WARNING

The difficulty with Level III devices is that technologists have no way to correct issues in real time if something goes wrong with the recording at home during the night. The only time technologists can check the quality of the recording is after the sleep study is completed and they receive the data.

Conducting the Level III sleep study

The lab staff may ask you to download an app on your smartphone that communicates with the recording electrodes or sensors you wear to collect the data during a Level III HST. In this case, you can follow these steps to conduct the sleep study:

1. **Apply your Level III device at bedtime according to the instructions you receive.**

See the preceding section for how you acquire the Level III device and instructions.

2. **Tap a button on the app you downloaded to start recording your sleep-related data.**

   You may need to disconnect and reconnect it if you get up during the night (for example, to use the bathroom).

3. **Go to sleep.**

4. **In the morning when you awaken, you may tap another button on the app to stop recording.**

5. **If prompted, follow the app instructions to transfer the data to the cloud.**

   Alternatively the data may simply remain in the device.

Depending on the Level III device you use, you have options for how to deal with the device after your successful sleep study. These include

REMEMBER

>> **Returning the device to the lab:** The lab may instruct you to return the device the next day. Or the lab may send you a message after receiving all of the data from the cloud; then you can return the device to the lab (often using a prepaid return box instead of returning it in person).

   Don't return the device unless lab staff has either pre-instructed you to return it the morning after the study or confirmed they have all the data they need (if the data transfers to the cloud).

>> **Dispose of a single-use device:** Some sleep laboratories use disposable, single-use devices. If that's the case for your study, you don't need to return the device at all. These devices come with instructions and an app for you to upload data to the cloud. The lab receives the study results, and you dispose of the device when they tell you to do so.

Receiving your HST results and diagnosis

After you conduct your at-home sleep study and return data to the lab, the technologists and sleep specialists review the results. You then receive an analysis of your results, a sleep disorder diagnosis, and next steps either via a message from the lab or at an in-person visit.

The main metric your specialist uses for diagnosing sleep apnea is the *apnea-hypopnea index* (AHI), which is the number of abnormal breathing events you experience divided by the hours of sleep you get. Consider these factors regarding the reliability of HST testing and diagnosis with Level III devices:

>> **Some devices don't accurately estimate sleep.** Instead, the devices use the total recording time in hours as the divisor (the denominator of the fraction

used to calculate the AHI), which includes times when you were not asleep. This results in a longer estimated amount of sleep time compared to the actual sleep time, which can dilute the AHI and underestimate the severity of sleep apnea.

>> **The sensitivity and specificity for detecting sleep apnea with home sleep tests are not as good as those in the lab (Level I studies).** Your Level III equipment might experience technical failures, or you might not use the device correctly. So if your HST doesn't show that you have sleep apnea, your sleep specialist may decide to order an in-laboratory study to make absolutely sure.

Using Actigraphy to Monitor Over Time

Actigraphy is a method sleep specialists use to monitor human rest and activity cycles. Typically, your sleep specialist has you wear a small device called an *actigraph*, which resembles a wristwatch that records movement through an accelerometer, typically in three axes (left–right, up–down, and forward–backward). Then your sleep specialist can analyze the data from the actigraph to help assess your sleep patterns and sleep–wake cycles of activity over extended periods.

Because patients can take actigraphs home and use them for two weeks or more, sleep specialists primarily use actigraphy to detect insomnia and circadian rhythm sleep disorders (to read more on these sleep disorders, turn to Chapter 7). Using an actigraph has these advantages; it offers

>> **An accurate view of sleep-wake patterns:** Measuring your sleep over a two-week period allows your specialist to get a very clear picture of habits, patterns, and behaviors — versus observing you for just one night in a sleep lab.

>> **Sleep related data as a precursor to other testing:** Your sleep specialist may also ask you to wear an actigraph for two weeks before you have an overnight in-laboratory sleep study, followed by a multiple sleep latency test (MSLT, an objective test of daytime sleepiness discussed in Chapter 7), so that the specialist can see whether you are having a consistent sleep-wake pattern before these other tests.

Comparing sleep data sources

Getting and wearing an actigraph

If your sleep specialist prescribes you actigraphy, you schedule a time to pick up the device at the sleep lab, where the technologist shows you how and when to wear it. Figure 10-5 shows an ActTrust 2, an actigraph device featured on the Condor Instruments website (https://condorinst.com/en/acttrust-two-actigraph).

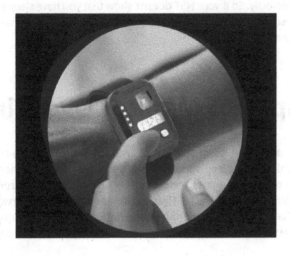

REMEMBER

Unless your doctor tells you otherwise, wear your actigraph for 24 hours a day — through the day and night. The only time you might be required to take it off is if you're bathing or swimming. Some actigraphs are actually waterproof or water resistant. Make sure that you know which kind you have.

Your sleep specialist will also ask you to keep track of your sleep-wake schedule by writing it in a sleep log or sleep diary during the 14 days or more that you're wearing the actigraph. Keeping a sleep log gives your sleep specialist a way to double-check when you go to bed, and when you wake up.

Some actigraphs have a light sensor that detects when you turn off your bedroom light and turn it back on, which gives a clue to your sleep specialist about when you settle down for the night. However, this technology is not foolproof, so the sleep log or diary allows your specialist to compare the sleep log data with the data from the actigraphy as a good secondary check.

Comparing sleep data sources

Together, the actigraphy and sleep logs provide a well-rounded night-to-night summary of your sleep schedule. Your provider can use these data to diagnose whether you have a certain circadian sleep-wake rhythm disorder or insomnia.

TIP

Comparing sleep logs to actigraphy is especially important in cases of insomnia because sleep logs alone aren't reliable. Sleep specialists can't be sure whether patients accurately convey their sleep periods because people suffering from insomnia often underestimate the amount of sleep they're getting, meaning that they often feel like they don't sleep at all during the night. But when the sleep specialist looks at the two weeks' worth of actigraphy data, they see the patient actually had different sleep periods throughout their 24-hour cycle. It might even amount to 6 or 7 hours of total sleep, but it's broken up over that 24-hour period, leading the patient to feel like they haven't slept.

Now, you might question why sleep labs use these actigraphy devices as opposed to consumer wearable health tracker devices, which assess sleep as well as other health domains such as activity, exercise, and diet. Two reasons for this are

» **Actigraphs are actual medical-grade devices**, meaning that they are typically FDA-approved for the specific purpose of monitoring sleep-wake cycles.

» **Many sleep labs and centers don't currently have a means of leveraging the data** from consumer wearable sleep tracker devices.

When providers need an objective look at their patients' sleep-wake cycles over an extended period of time, actigraphy is the answer. However, consumer health trackers are rapidly developing over time, and it's not inconceivable that eventually they will replace conventional actigraphy.

Other Technology and Testing Methods

Sleep specialists have other technological devices and testing methods that they can use to evaluate sleep and wakefulness in various settings. These include

» **The *psychomotor vigilance task* (PVT),** a test that gives your specialist the ability to estimate a patient's *sustained attention* (the ability to focus for a long period of time in the presence of other distractions). It is primarily used in research settings, but a provider may use the PVT to objectively test how alert or vigilant you are during the daytime as an alternative to the maintenance of wakefulness test in the laboratory. The test assesses sleepiness- or fatigue-related changes in alertness and is sensitive to the effects of sleep loss or deprivation, or to circadian rhythm sleep-wake disorders. You can perform this PVT test using an app on your phone or a device from the lab. You start the device (or app) and are instructed to respond to a visual signal on the device by pressing a key. This tests your reaction time, which is a good surrogate marker for alertness. Your specialist may instruct you to use this app several times throughout the day.

>> **The Oxford Sleep Resistance test (OSLER),** which sleep specialists also use in research settings. Similar to the PVT, this test assesses your ability to maintain alertness. You hit a button placed on a box directly connected to a computer when you see a visual stimulus that appears every few seconds.

>> **The CPAP, BPAP, ASV, and AVAPS devices,** which are all smart devices that have SD or other memory cards and the ability to transfer data to the cloud. These features enable the devices to collect sleep and sleep-related breathing data during the night and make these data available to the prescribing sleep specialist. The specialists can obtain data remotely, including data such as apnea-hypopnea index (AHI), air leak, device use per night, and percentage of use over time.

Sleep specialists can even remotely adjust the setting of these devices, such as increasing or decreasing the pressures. But the devices themselves can also adjust the pressures within a prescribed range to allow the minimum amount of air pressure during the night in order to keep the upper airway open and minimize abnormal sleep-related breathing events.

Chapter 11

Using Wearables, Nearables, and Airables, Oh My!

S leep is crucial to your health, but understanding how well you sleep can be tricky. Fortunately, rapidly advancing technology makes tracking your sleep patterns to optimize your rest easy to do. Devices such as smartwatches, under-mattress sensors, and even your phone's microphone provide detailed data on how long you sleep, how often you wake up, and whether you're experiencing conditions such as sleep apnea.

Many consumer health trackers incorporate technology to track overall health and fitness, specific health measures (such as cardiac rate and blood pressure), nutrition, and other indices, including sleep. However, I exclusively focus on the sleep technology of these devices and refer to them as consumer sleep trackers even though they might also include these other measures.

In this chapter, I show you how sleep-tracking technology — including wearables, nearables, and airables — helps you understand and take control of your sleep habits and problems. Whether you're wearing a wristband that monitors your heart rate or placing a sensor under your mattress, the data you collect gives you insights that formerly were available only through clinical sleep studies. You can find out how each type of device works, how accurate they are, and how they compare to traditional medical approaches such as polysomnography (PSG, used in a sleep lab; see Chapter 10). Plus, you discover the practicalities and precautions that come with using electronics to monitor your sleep.

Sleeping with a Tracker

Tracking your sleep is simpler than ever. After the COVID-19 pandemic of 2020, consumer sleep-tracking devices are more available, and the public demonstrates increased interest not only in general health but also in sleep health. Some research (by LinkedIn, for example) estimates that the consumer sleep tracking devices market is expected to grow to $57.97 billion USD by 2030.

With a variety of these devices on the market, soon you may no longer need to visit a sleep clinic to understand your nightly habits. Instead, you can slip on a smart-watch, place a sensor under your mattress, or even use the microphone on your phone to track your sleep. These consumer sleep trackers are split into these three categories:

>> **Wearables** are the most common and familiar tracking devices think Fitbit or Apple Watch. You wear them on your body, usually your wrist, and they track everything from how long you sleep to your heart rate and oxygen levels.

>> **Nearables** are devices that you don't wear but that stay close to you — for example, under-mattress sensors. You just set them up, and they work in the background while you sleep.

>> **Airables** are the newest category. They use wireless signals, such as radio waves, sounds, or sonar, to monitor your sleep. Airables may already be part of your life and home environment in the form of smart home devices like your virtual assistant.

The distinction between nearables and airables is a bit controversial, since some scientists argue that the dividing line between these two categories is blurry and the devices within the airable category might really fit within the nearable category.

REMEMBER

Some devices are hybrids of these tracker categories; for example, an app that monitors sound via the smartphone's microphone demonstrates an airable func-tionality. But the same app can sense motion via the smartphone's placement on the mattress, which demonstrates a nearable feature. The sound and motions work together to estimate sleep parameters.

TIP

Each device offers different features for collecting data about your sleep, and with multiple types of devices on the market, you can choose the type (or types) that works best for your lifestyle.

Knowing what consumer sleep trackers track

Consumer sleep trackers (as well as in-laboratory sleep studies and home sleep tests) typically report sleep parameters and sleep-related events, as outlined in Table 11-1. Some devices may also have a proprietary type of *sleep score*, which is a device-specific assessment of sleep quality.

TABLE 11-1 **Sleep Parameters and Events**

Sleep Parameters and Sleep-Related Events	Descriptions
Time in bed (TIB)	Amount of time in bed from bedtime (lights off) to wake time (lights on)
Total sleep time (TST), time asleep, sleep duration	Total amount of time asleep
Sleep period time (SPT)	Amount of time between sleep onset (first two consecutive min of N2, N3, or REM sleep) and the end of sleep (the last two consecutive min of N1, N2, N3, or REM sleep)
Sleep onset (SO)	Clock time (hrs:min:sec; for example 10:12:02) of the onset of sleep
Sleep latency (SL) or sleep onset latency (SOL)	Amount of time between bedtime (lights off) to sleep onset
Sleep efficiency (SE)	Amount of time spent asleep divided by the time in bed expressed as a percentage: (TST/TIB) x 100
Sleep cycle	Amount of time elapsed during different stages of sleep (light/deep/REM sleep)
Sleep-time difference	Average sleep duration on weekends minus the average sleep duration on weekdays; this difference represents the total amount of extra sleep typically obtained on weekends when compared to weekdays
REM sleep latency	Amount of time from sleep onset to the first REM period
REM sleep time	Amount of rapid eye movement (REM) sleep
Bedtime	Clock time (hrs:min:sec) for bedtime (lights off)
Wake time	Clock time (hrs:min:sec) for final awakening when arising from bed (lights off)

(continued)

TABLE 11-1 *(continued)*

Sleep Parameters and Sleep-Related Events	Descriptions
Wake after sleep onset (WASO)	Amount of time awake between sleep onset to final awakening
Sleep fragmentation/ arousal index	Number of fragmentation/arousals per hour of sleep
Light sleep or N1/N2 time	Amount of time in light (N1/N2) sleep
Deep sleep or N3 time	Amount of time in deep (N3) sleep
Snoring	The frequency, intensity, and/or duration of snoring may be reported
Respiratory disturbance index (RDI)	A less used index (versus the AHI) that includes the number of apneas, hypopneas, and respiratory effort–related arousals (RERAs, brief awakenings of sleep caused by slowed breathing that doesn't meet criteria for apneas or hypopneas) per hour of sleep
Apnea-hypopnea index (AHI)	Number of apneas and hypopneas per hour of sleep (see Chapter 8 for additional details)
Oxygen desaturation index (ODI)	Number of oxygen desaturation episodes, defined as a decrease in the mean oxygen saturation of ≥3% or ≥4% (over the last 120 seconds) that lasts for at least 10 seconds
Minimum oxygen saturation	Lowest oxygen saturation level during the recorded period
Periodic limb movements index (PLMI)	Number of periodic limb movements per hour of sleep (see Chapter 8 for further explanation). PLMAI, which are the number of arousals (brief awakenings) per hour of sleep associated with periodic limb movements are also calculated
Heart rate	The average, minimum, and maximum heart rate during wakefulness and sleep stages are often calculated, in addition to noting any cardiac arrhythmias
Body Position	The time spent in different body positions (left, right, prone, supine) are indicated, as well as the amount/percent of time of stages of sleep and breathing parameters (AHI)

Assessing sleep-tracker data versus sleep-lab data

Consumer sleep trackers are convenient and easy to use, but their accuracy depends on the technology behind them and the specific device. Although these devices have improved over the years, they still aren't as precise as *polysomnography* (PSG, sleep study that you get in a sleep laboratory, which is the gold-standard test for monitoring sleep). Even with PSG, however, sleep experts generally agree only around 85 percent of the time when determining the different stages of the sleep-wake cycle (wake, N1, N2, N3, and REM).

When comparing sleep trackers to PSG, you have three key metrics to consider:

>> **Sensitivity:** How well the device identifies actual sleep

Currently, compared to PSG, most consumer trackers tend to overestimate total sleep time and underestimate wake after sleep onset (how much time you spend awake after falling asleep).

>> **Specificity:** How well the device identifies actual wakefulness

Consumer trackers are generally good at detecting sleep (high sensitivity), but only moderately good at detecting wakefulness (specificity).

>> **Accuracy:** How well a device identifies both sleep and wake correctly overall

WARNING

For people with sleep disorders, these trackers are less accurate, probably because the disorder affects sleep patterns and quality. Also, accuracy tends to vary with the user's age — for example, by giving more inconsistent readings for adolescents.

Taking advantage of wearable devices

Wearable devices are the most popular consumer sleep trackers, and they've come a long way since Fitbit first introduced sleep-tracking in the early 2010s. These devices monitor your sleep — primarily through motion-based tracking — by using accelerometers to detect when you move and multi-sensor tracking to differentiate between wake and various sleep stages. Specifically, this multi-sensor tracking combines motion data with heart rate and heart rate variability derived from *photoplethysmography* (PPG, a non-invasive technology that measures blood volume changes in the skin by the amount of light absorbed by tissues, blood, and blood vessels). See the section "Assessing Sleep Conditions with Technology" later in the chapter for more information.

TIP

Wearables are a great option for tracking your sleep because their advancements can now monitor multiple sleep-related metrics. Unlike traditional *actigraphy* (a wristwatch-like device which uses accelerometers that detect motion to estimate sleep-wake patterns), many consumer sleep trackers offer more sophisticated technology. Actigraphy is typically used by sleep specialists to diagnose circadian rhythm disorders (see Chapter 10 for more on this), but it often lacks the technology that consumer devices now offer. Plus, the cost and insurance limitations of actigraphy have been a limiting factor for their use in sleep medicine.

Wearable devices come in various forms:

» **Wristbands:** Smartwatches like the Fitbit or Apple Watch are common examples of devices that assess sleep. Figure 11-1 (on the left) shows a Fitbit Charge 6, as sold on Amazon (www.amazon.com).

» **Rings:** Smart rings — like the Oura Ring 4 shown in Figure 11-1 (on the right) as sold at Best Buy (www.bestbuy.com) — track heart rate variability and temperature. The smart ring is a great option if you don't like to wear anything on your wrist.

» **Headbands:** Some wearable devices are designed to be worn on your head to track brain activity during sleep. Figure 11-2 depicts a Muse S Headband as sold on the Muse website (https://choosemuse.com).

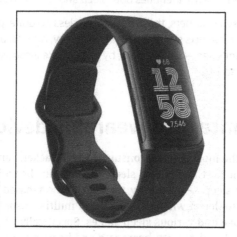 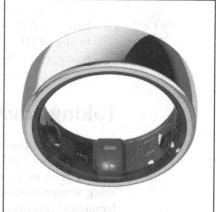

FIGURE 11-1:
A Fitbit device (left) and an Oura smart ring (right).

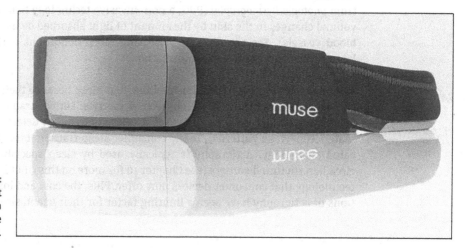

FIGURE 11-2:
A headband that tracks brain activity while you sleep.

These devices can also track additional metrics such as breathing patterns, oxygen levels, and even body temperature, which makes them a comprehensive tool for sleep monitoring.

Table 11-2 lists both advantages and potential drawbacks of using wearables to track sleep.

TABLE 11-2 ## Advantages and Drawbacks of Wearables

Advantages	
Wearable Devices Are	What It Means
Multifunctional	Wearables track more than just sleep; they can monitor fitness, heart rate, daily activity, and risk for sleep disorders such as obstructive sleep apnea.
Convenient	Lightweight and worn throughout the day and night, wearables offer 24-hour monitoring.
Accurate	Many wearable devices have significantly improved in estimating sleep stages and overall sleep quality.
Potential Drawbacks	
Wearable Devices Can	What It Means
Cause discomfort	Wearing a device while sleeping may feel uncomfortable or may disrupt your sleep.
Overestimate sleep	Wearables may overestimate sleep by interpreting long periods of stillness as sleep because (unlike PSG) they don't use brain wave patterns (as well as eye movements and muscle activity) to directly measure sleep.

Getting close with nearables

Nearables, such as under-mattress sensors, offer an excellent alternative if you'd rather not wear something while you sleep. These devices work passively and monitor your sleep without needing to be attached to your body. After you install a nearable device under your mattress, it can capture data on your sleep-wake patterns — such as total sleep time and wake periods — by detecting subtle movements through the mattress.

Nearables have notable benefits:

>> **No physical attachment:** You don't need to wear anything on your body, which eliminates discomfort.

>> **Long-term monitoring:** Many nearable devices allow you to track data over weeks, months, or even years, which provides a comprehensive view of your sleep patterns.

>> **Detection of sleep-disordered breathing:** Nearables have proven to be effective in detecting conditions such as sleep-disordered breathing.

Examples of nearable devices include

>> **Withings Sleep Tracking Mat:** A mat that slips under your mattress to monitor sleep cycles, heart rate, and breathing.

>> **Sleeptracker-AI:** An under-mattress device that tracks sleep and detects sleep-disordered breathing. Figure 11-3 shows the Sleeptracker AI, which is depicted on the Sleeptracker website (https://sleeptracker.com).

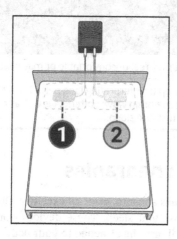 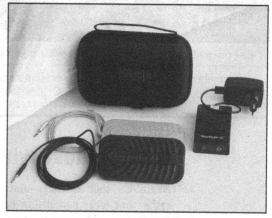

FIGURE 11-3:
Under mattress sensors are unobtrusive and allow unencumbered sleeping.

REMEMBER

Nearables, although they offer a contactless solution, may be affected by external factors such as the type of mattress you use or the presence of other movements in the bed. For example, if you sleep with a partner or a pet, their movements may have the potential of influencing the data collected by the under-mattress sensors (although these devices have algorithms for detecting these extraneous movements).

Opting for airables

Airable devices might sound like something out of science fiction, but they're already here. These devices, such as a smartphone app called *Sleep Routine*, use wireless signals to monitor your sleep. By detecting sound or bouncing radio waves off your body, they detect movement and breathing patterns without physical contact. Airables work by using the microphone on your phone or a bedside device to collect the data, which makes them incredibly easy to set up.

Figure 11-4 shows how you can use a smartphone's microphone in combination with an app to track sleep patterns, providing a convenient, no-contact solution. In this case, the app is AsleepTrack API, whose monitoring features are depicted on the Asleep website (https://www.asleep.ai/en/product).

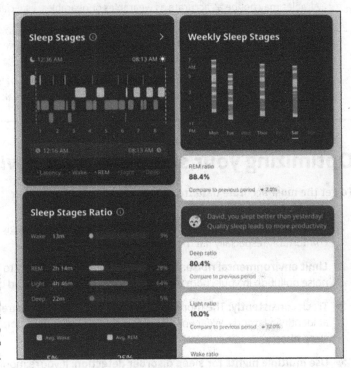

FIGURE 11-4:
An airable device using a smartphone's microphone to monitor sleep and breathing.

Airable devices offer several key benefits and also some less-than-perfect characteristics, as listed in Table 11-3.

TABLE 11-3　　**Benefits and Downsides of Airable Devices**

Benefits	
What It Is	**Description**
No specialized hardware required	You need only a smart device, which you may already own — such as smartphone or a smart device such as Amazon Echo.
Ease of use	Airables require no setup beyond downloading an app or enabling a feature on your smart device.
Cost-effectiveness	Because most airables rely on existing hardware, they may be cheaper than wearables or nearables.
Downsides	
What It Is	**Description**
Accuracy	Airables may not be as accurate as wearables or nearables, especially for detecting smaller movements or more detailed sleep stages.
Multiple features	Airable apps may offer fewer health metrics when compared to wearables and nearables.
Vulnerability	Airables are subject to environmental interference because they rely on sound or radio waves. Background noises, poor microphone quality, or weak signals can all impact device effectiveness.

Optimizing your sleep-tracking device

To get the most accurate data from your consumer sleep tracker

>> **Wear your device properly:** Make sure your wearable fits snugly but comfortably, especially if it monitors heart rate and breathing.

>> **Limit environmental noise:** If you're using airable devices, try to minimize noise pollution in your room to improve the quality of the sound data.

>> **Track consistently:** The more data your device collects, the better it becomes at identifying trends. Wear your tracker nightly to build up a comprehensive sleep history.

>> **Use multiple nights for sleep disorder detection:** If you're monitoring for sleep apnea or other disorders, rely on data from several nights instead of a single night's reading. Studies show that tracking over multiple nights improves the accuracy of identifying conditions such as obstructive sleep apnea (OSA).

Assessing Sleep Conditions with Technology

Sleep-tracking devices aren't just for monitoring how many hours you sleep. They also help you assess more serious conditions such as sleep apnea, where your breathing repeatedly stops and starts throughout the night (if you want to read more about sleep apnea, turn to Chapter 7). Consumer sleep trackers detect sleep, sleep apnea, and circadian rhythm sleep-wake problems by using

WARNING

>> **Pulse oximetry:** Devices measure blood oxygen levels to determine whether you experience dips (decreases in these levels) during the night — a situation that can indicate sleep apnea.

   Pulse oximetry can be less accurate and overestimate oxygen saturation for individuals with darker skin tones because skin pigmentation can interfere with the readings. The same issue can occur when an individual is wearing nail polish and using a device that clips over the finger. Device developers are working to address this issue, but consider this factor if you're relying on these devices for health insights.

>> **Breathing rate tracking:** Some wearables and nearables monitor your breathing patterns to detect irregularities like apneas or hypopneas.

>> **Heart rate variability (HRV):** Changes in HRV can signal disruptions in sleep caused by sleep-related breathing disorders. Heart rate is higher and HRV is lower during wake compared to sleep. Devices can also estimate HRV by taking acoustic measurements, such as tracheal breath sounds.

>> **Photoplethysmography (PPG):** Measures the amount of light absorbed by tissues, blood, and blood vessels, Wavelengths of light differ in their ability to penetrate deeper tissue (for example, red light can reach deeper into tissue than can green light). Tracking devices use PPG signals to detect variations such as blood volume, blood pressure, oxygen saturation, and pulse rate.

>> **Peripheral arterial tonometry (PAT):** Uses optical sensors to measure arterial pulse volume changes in the finger as a result of vasomotion (*vasoconstriction* and *vasodilatation*, the narrowing and widening of blood vessels). PAT can detect respiratory events characteristic of sleep apnea and also cardiovascular risk factors.

>> **Ballistocardiography (BCG):** Assesses body motion produced by the ejection of the blood at each cardiac cycle. The BCG technology involves *accelerometers* (devices that measure vibration or change in motion) and *micro-bend fiber optic sensors* (MFOS, a small bend in optical fibers to measure physical parameters). Also, materials that produce an electrical charge in response

to an applied mechanical stress — piezoelectric sensors or electromechanical film — can detect BCG signals. These signals are also used frequently to monitor breathing during sleep.

>> **Cardiopulmonary coupling (CPC):** Links heart and respiration rates to assess sleep-related parameters. CPC analysis can use a variety of signals, including those from electrocardiograms (ECGs), photoplethysmograms (PPGs), and blood pressure monitors.

TIP

If your sleep tracker shows irregularities in breathing or oxygen levels, consult a healthcare provider to assess whether you may have a sleep disorder such as obstructive sleep apnea (OSA).

HELPING SLEEP DISORDERS WITH CONSUMER SLEEP TRACKERS

People use a variety of consumer devices to provide remedies or treatments for sleep problems and disorders. Such devices include

- Mobile cognitive behavioral treatment for insomnia (CBT-I)

- Apps that prompt daily orofacial myofunctional therapy (OMT) exercises to strengthen the upper airway muscles, a practice that may improve obstructive sleep apnea (OSA)

- A headband that delivers acoustic resonance therapy to improve sleep quality

- Leg-worn devices that deliver mild electrical stimulation and improve symptoms of restless legs syndrome (RLS)

- Head-worn devices that produce transcranial electrical stimulation to improve sleep and clearance of metabolic waste products in the brain

Currently, types of devices that focus more on therapies for sleep problems and disorders are much less common than sleep trackers. But with the omnipresence of consumer sleep trackers, manufacturers will likely develop more of these therapeutic devices that — when coupled with sleep trackers — can provide both assessment and therapy solutions.

Tracking sleep to identify OSA

With around 1 billion people worldwide affected by obstructive sleep apnea (OSA) — including approximately 54 million in the U.S. alone — sleep-tracking devices are likely to become even more useful in the future. Of those millions in the U.S., around 43 million are thought to have OSA that is untreated.

Smartwatches like those from Samsung and Apple are already helping detect the risk of OSA in people who wear them. Patients now commonly bring sleep data from their smartphones to their healthcare providers, a practice that helps with diagnosis and treatment discussions.

TIP

If you know someone who regularly complains about poor sleep but resists seeing a doctor, you can suggest that they try wearing a sleep-tracking device. Sleep trackers can increase awareness of sleep patterns and disorders, especially in people who might be at risk for conditions such as OSA. The data they gather could encourage them to seek medical help sooner.

Looking for circadian rhythm disorders

In addition to detecting sleep apnea, consumer sleep trackers can help identify circadian rhythm sleep-wake disorders. These devices collect data over many days and nights, which helps reveal disrupted sleep-wake patterns over time. Like they do with medical-grade actigraphy tracking, sleep specialists may be able to use the information from consumer sleep trackers when diagnosing circadian rhythm sleep-wake disorders. For more information on these disorders, flip to Chapter 7.

Facing the challenges of tracking sleep disorders with consumer devices

Consumer sleep trackers aren't perfect, and users face several challenges when using the trackers to find and offer data related to sleep disorders. For example, you have

>> **Lack of cohesive reporting:** The many different devices don't share a common IT platform for data integration and display.

>> **Missing connection with electronic health record systems:** These devices currently can't integrate into the electronic health record systems of hospitals and clinics.

>> **Difficulty in discerning relevant data:** Consumer devices provide a vast amount of data, and clinicians, researchers, and users find that deciding on which data are most relevant and useful is difficult to do.

- >> **Concentration on the wellness market:** Manufacturers of these devices also may want to stay in the large consumer wellness space rather than venture into the increasingly competitive area of medical-grade devices that must meet FDA requirements for the diagnosis of sleep disorders, such as obstructive sleep apnea.

- >> **Proprietary algorithms that mask raw data:** Many of the consumer sleep trackers use proprietary algorithms for assessment of sleep and sleep-disordered breathing, which prevents users from sharing raw and scored sleep data with their clinicians. And thus clinicians can feel that the devices use a *black box approach* (a methodology that is hidden from the user) and lack transparency.

- >> **Lack of data examining diverse populations:** The numbers of research studies exploring and testing new devices are increasing dramatically, but few studies examine different clinical populations outside of the controlled sleep laboratory setting. In addition, data that assesses patients with OSA-related comorbidities (such as obesity, hypertension, cardiovascular disease, and diabetes) is lacking for consumer sleep-tracking devices.

Taking Precautions When Using Electronics for Sleep Tracking

Using a sleep-tracker device can offer valuable insights, but you must stay mindful of the potential downsides. The *quantified self movement* is all about using technology to track your daily life to improve your physical, mental, and emotional well-being. And although gathering data on your sleep can be helpful, becoming overly focused on the numbers can backfire. A condition known as *orthosomnia* can happen when you obsess so much over perfecting your sleep that this behavior and accompanying stress can actually create more sleep problems.

WARNING

Constantly checking your phone for sleep data, especially in the middle of the night, disrupts your sleep. The blue light from your screen can interfere with your circadian sleep-wake rhythm, and the act of looking at your phone can wake up your brain and make falling back asleep more difficult. Remember, sleep trackers are tools to help you, not to stress you out!

TIP

To prevent orthosomnia, try

>> **Setting a limit on checking your data:** Avoid looking at your sleep data first thing in the morning or right before bed.

>> **Using a blue light filter:** If you must check your phone, use a filter to reduce blue light exposure.

>> **Keeping your phone somewhere other than on the bed:** Charge your phone away from your bed to resist the urge to check it during the night.

>> **Discussing tracking with your child's pediatrician:** If children or teens are using sleep-tracking devices, ensure that they are using them responsibly, especially because young users are prone to over-checking of and dependency on data.

Despite these challenges, given the ubiquity of wearable, nearable, and airable devices and the growing interest from the public, consumer sleep trackers are here to stay and will become even more firmly entrenched in the future of sleep and sleep medicine.

Chapter 12

Looking Toward the Future for Better Sleep Health

The future holds exciting possibilities for improving sleep health and for the management of sleep disorders. Sleep diagnostics and treatments have come a long way from where they started (to read about the evolution and notable moments in the history of sleep medicine, turn to Chapter 2), and the future holds even more promise.

Imagine a world in which your mattress adjusts its firmness based on your sleep patterns or a simple wearable device predicts a sleepless night before it happens. Sounds like science fiction, doesn't it? It's closer to reality than you might think. The sleep tech revolution is here, and it transforms how we understand and manage sleep. Whether you battle sleep apnea, restless legs syndrome, or insomnia, staying informed about these emerging technologies can make all the difference in tackling your issue.

In this chapter, I dive into the latest advancements that transform the way sleep specialists diagnose and treat sleep disorders. You get a sneak peek at the cutting-edge developments that can shape the future of sleep health. From AI-driven sleep plans to gene therapy, the innovations on the horizon are truly mind-blowing.

Enhancing Sleep and Tackling Sleep Disorders

Medical engineers and researchers have exciting innovations currently in development that are aimed at helping you achieve better sleep. Emerging consumer technologies — such as smart mattresses, wearable sleep trackers, and advanced noise-canceling devices — pave the way for a more restful night's sleep.

If you look ahead to the next five years, you can anticipate that several consumer-level sleep aids may become more mainstream, more personalized, and full-service. These devices will not only track your sleep, but also provide you with customized recommendations to improve your sleep quality.

TIP

By staying informed about developments in sleep-aid technology and considering innovative treatments, you can take proactive steps towards achieving better sleep health. These advancements highlight a future where sleep disorders are no longer a chronic struggle, but a condition that specialists can effectively treat and even cure.

Invoking sleep-conducive surroundings

One possible sleep aid involves the integration of artificial intelligence (AI) with smart home systems to help create a sleep-friendly environment. Imagine a system that dims the lights, adjusts the thermostat, and plays soothing sounds that prepare you for sleep — based on your tracked sleep data. Additionally, advancements in neurotechnology could lead to wearable devices that stimulate your brain waves to promote deeper sleep or shorten the time you need to fall asleep. As technologies like these evolve, they promise to make achieving a good night's sleep easier and more personalized.

Other sleep-centered innovations include

» **Sleep pods** (structures or chairs in which people can take a private nap) are another sleep aid that's becoming increasingly popular in some workplaces and airports. They may also soon appear in other public spaces to provide convenient napping options.

» **Sleep tourism** (a practice in which you travel to destinations that offer specialized sleep programs) is also on the rise. Many hotels are taking an increasingly serious approach to prioritizing sleep by working with sleep centers to optimize their rooms to create a sleep-inducing environment.

>> ***Sleep-sensitive scheduling*** for schools and businesses that recognizes sleep patterns. Educators and employers have a growing awareness of how sleep impacts productivity and learning. Many schools and workplaces across the U.S. continue to adjust their schedules to better align with natural sleep patterns.

REMEMBER

Later school start times for adolescents and flexible work hours for adults can help improve overall sleep quality and daytime performance for both groups.

Treating sleep issues with clinical advancements

On a clinical level, advancements in medical research and technology are revolutionizing how sleep professionals understand and treat sleep disorders. Exciting developments in this area include the use of

>> ***Gene therapy*** (a medical technique for modifying a person's genes as treatment) to tackle sleep issues at their root cause. By targeting specific genes associated with sleep disorders, researchers are working on therapies that can potentially cure conditions such as insomnia and narcolepsy. This approach goes beyond symptom management and aims for a long-term solution that addresses the underlying genetic factors.

>> ***Neuromodulation,*** a technique that involves using electrical or magnetic stimulation to regulate the nervous system, thereby improving sleep patterns. For individuals with conditions such as restless legs syndrome (RLS) or insomnia, neuromodulation offers a new and effective treatment option. By directly influencing the brain's activity, it can help normalize sleep rhythms and reduce the symptoms that disrupt your sleep. I talk more about stimulation treatments in the section "Diagnosing and treating specific sleep disorders" later in the chapter.

>> ***Pharmacogenomics*** — a field that studies how your genetic makeup affects your response to different medications — is opening up new possibilities for tailored, personalized treatments. By understanding genetic influences, doctors can prescribe sleep medications specifically suited to your body's needs, which can increase their effectiveness and reduce potential side effects. This personalized approach ensures that you receive the most effective treatment for your unique condition, paving the way for better management of sleep disorders.

Emerging Technologies in the Sleep Field

In the rapidly evolving field of sleep medicine, emerging technologies are reshaping how specialists diagnose and treat sleep disorders. From new imaging techniques to innovative treatments, technological developments are providing new hope and solutions for sleep-related issues.

Artificial intelligence (AI)

Artificial intelligence (AI) is poised to revolutionize sleep diagnostics and bring new levels of accuracy and efficiency to the field. Future diagnostic advancements will likely harness AI's capability to analyze vast amounts of data and provide real-time insights. This capability can transform how sleep professionals diagnose and treat sleep disorders.

For example, AI can provide

>> **Advanced real-time note-taking:** Future AI systems will go beyond current capabilities, providing even more accurate and comprehensive notes during medical visits, reducing the need for manual transcription.

>> **Advanced sleep pattern analysis:** AI algorithms will evolve to detect more subtle patterns and anomalies in your sleep data that might not be apparent through current observation methods.

>> **Highly personalized sleep plans:** By integrating data from even more diverse sources, AI will create highly tailored sleep improvement plans, offering specific advice on bedtime routines, diet, and exercise that is uniquely suited to each individual.

>> **Enhanced MRI and CT scan analysis:** Future applications of AI may include even more sophisticated analysis of MRI and CT scans of the upper airway, offering detailed insights into potential obstructions or abnormalities with greater accuracy.

>> **Enhanced presumed diagnosis:** AI will be able to provide more precise preliminary diagnoses by deeply analyzing physicians' notes and patient symptoms, helping doctors identify potential issues even faster and more accurately.

REMEMBER

AI can assist in early symptom detection, providing valuable insights for proactive treatment.

>> **Predictive analytics in sleep apps:** Future apps will leverage AI to offer predictive analytics, allowing them to anticipate and prevent sleep disordered episodes before they occur. These technologies can analyze extensive data

from your sleep patterns and predict disruptions, offering real-time adjustments to your sleep environment or schedule to enhance sleep quality.

>> **Predictive health monitoring:** Future AI will predict potential sleep issues with greater accuracy, allowing for proactive measures to be taken well before issues become problematic.

TIP

Consistently use the AI tools that are at your disposal to help stay ahead of sleep issues and maintain better overall health. Your related benefits include personalized insights from diagnostic efforts and proactive health management — both of which can ensure better sleep quality and overall well-being.

Machine learning (ML)

Machine learning (ML) is set to significantly enhance the field of sleep diagnostics by improving the reliability and efficiency of sleep studies. Future ML advancements aim to analyze biosignals from both home sleep tests and laboratory studies. The goal is to enable better recognition of sleep stages and the detection of abnormalities such as breathing disorders and periodic limb movements.

Look for emerging developments such as

>> **Advanced detection of abnormalities:** Upcoming ML algorithms will detect a wider range of sleep abnormalities, including more precise identification of apneas, hypopneas, leg movements, and heart rhythm irregularities, processing vast amounts of data even more quickly.

>> **Broader integration:** As these algorithms advance, they will become more widely integrated into sleep labs, further enhancing the diagnostic process and offering more reliable results for patients.

>> **Continued improvement in reliability:** ML algorithms will continue to improve, potentially exceeding the reliability of current manual scoring with significantly higher interrater reliability for sleep stage detection.

>> **Efficiency in sleep labs:** Future ML algorithms will enhance the scoring process even further, providing more consistent and reliable scoring, significantly reducing the need for manual review by technologists and physicians. These algorithms will reduce interrater variability and improve diagnostic accuracy.

REMEMBER

By incorporating advanced ML algorithms, future sleep labs can offer more consistent and accurate diagnoses that minimize the potential for human error.

>> **Enhanced sleep stage recognition:** Future ML algorithms will analyze sleep stages with even greater reliability than current methods, further reducing the time it takes to score sleep studies and increasing efficiency in sleep labs. This will enhance the recognition of sleep stages and abnormalities, including apneas, hypopneas, and periodic limb movements.

TIP

Staying informed about these technologies can allow you to take proactive steps to improve your sleep health.

Diagnosing and treating specific sleep disorders

New and emerging technologies are enhancing the accuracy and comfort of diagnosing and treating sleep-related breathing disorders, sleep-related movement disorders, parasomnias, circadian rhythm sleep-wake disorders, hypersomnias, and insomnia. The innovations aim to improve patient experience and pinpoint

>> **The exact location of airway obstructions and more customized treatments** for an obstructive sleep apnea sufferer

>> **More precise detection and less invasive treatment solutions** for those who have sleep-related movement disorders such as restless legs syndrome (RLS), periodic limb movement disorder (PLMD), and sleep-related rhythmic movement disorder

>> **Methods for detecting abnormal sleep-wake rhythms and restoring regular sleep patterns** for patients who have circadian rhythm sleep-wake disorders

>> **Detecting and controlling unusual nighttime behaviors** in the home environment (for patients who experience parasomnias)

>> **Ways to improve sleep, daily functioning, and quality of life** for hypersomnia patients

>> **Methods for detecting sleep and for improving sleep quality and overall health outcomes** for those with insomnia

Tables 12-1 through 12-6 offer an outline of the technological advances related to the diagnosis and treatment of these various sleep disorders.

Regarding technology advancements for breathing disorders such as OSA, the DISE diagnostic (see Table 12-1) is effective, but may not be available in all regions of the U.S. If you've tried CPAP therapy but it didn't help, hypoglossal nerve stimulation might be the solution that works for you!

TABLE 12-1   Obstructive Sleep Apnea Advancements

Diagnosis Technology	How It Works
Drug-Induced Sleep Endoscopy (DISE)	Employs light sedation and a sleep surgeon inserts a tiny camera called a *nasopharyngeal endoscope* into your nose to look for obstructions in your upper airway; this procedure is becoming more commonly used.
Ultrasound	Requires no sedation and visualizes your upper airway through noninvasive scans; this is an emerging technology.
Endotyping (classifying diseases into subtypes based on their underlying biological mechanisms)	Methods that are not yet in widespread use to classify OSA into subtypes based on underlying causes, such as a narrowed upper airway, weakness of airway dilator muscles, fluid shift from legs to head and neck while sleeping, decreased lung volume, low arousal threshold, and loop gain (unstable breathing). Further research is expected to offer more personalized management for these OSA endotypes.

Treatment Development	How It Works
Medications	Development of medications to improve muscle activity in the upper airway (atomoxetine and oxybutynin) and treat obesity (tirzepatide).
External devices and implants	Create back pressure toward the upper airway to keep it open during exhalation by using devices such as external nasal valves, applying external pressure to the neck by collars to open the airway, and opening the nasal passages by nasal stents.
Hypoglossal nerve stimulation	A pacemaker-like implant under the skin on your chest that detects your breathing pattern and connects to the hypoglossal nerve in the tongue to deliver a mild electrical stimulation that moves the tongue forward to keep the airway open.
Positional therapy	Helps you maintain a side-sleeping position by using devices such as inflatable pillows or belts with sensors that use gentle sounds or vibrations to alert you when you roll onto your back, since OSA is typically worse when lying on your back.
Phrenic nerve stimulation	Monitors respiratory signals during sleep and stimulates the phrenic nerve to move the diaphragm and restore normal breathing, which is a promising alternative to *adaptive servo-ventilation* (ASV) devices used for central sleep apnea treatment.

REMEMBER

Positional therapy treatment devices can sometimes cause sleep disturbances because the stimuli that certain devices use may cause you to have a brief awakening. The awakening is not long or strong enough to fully wake you up, but it might fragment your sleep. Make sure to consult your doctor before you try positional therapy devices.

TABLE 12-2   Sleep-Related Movement Disorders

Diagnosis	
Technology	**How It Works**
Wearable devices	Employ advanced motion sensors and AI to continuously monitor and analyze leg movements throughout the night to provide data on frequency and intensity of these movements in order to aid in the characterization and diagnosis of periodic limb movement disorder (PLMD)
Non-invasive neural interfaces	Aim to detect neurological signals associated with sleep-related movements and to provide a clearer picture of the brain's role in the causes of these movements for more tailored treatment approaches

Treatment	
Development	**How It Works**
Vibration pads	Stimulates the skin receptors in the legs with the promise of relieving symptoms in the future
Nerve stimulation	Stimulates the legs and *peroneal nerve* (which provides sensation and movement to the foot, toes, and lower leg) with bands and other devices that apply electrical stimulation, pressure, or massage to calm restless legs
Vestibular (inner ear) stimulation	Rocks the bed to provide vestibular stimulation for individuals with sleep-related rhythmic movement disorder to help manage symptoms and induce sleep

TIP

For the treatment of sleep-related movement disorders, pads, bands, and rocking-bed stimuli are particularly beneficial because they offer a non-drug solution that may help to alleviate your symptoms without the side effects associated with medications.

TABLE 12-3   Circadian Rhythm Sleep-Wake Disorders

Diagnosis	
Technology	**How It Works**
Consumer wearable, airable, and nearable devices	Enable individuals to monitor their sleep-wake cycles and spot potential circadian rhythm sleep-wake disorders outside of the lab.
Biosensors in consumer wearables devices	Continuously monitor physiological parameters (such as your heart rate) associated with circadian rhythm sleep-wake disorders and provide real-time data.
Dim-light melatonin onset (DLMO) *assays* (tests that determine ingredients)	Patients take periodic saliva samples — which sleep specialists can analyze to create a melatonin profile to assist in the diagnosis of specific circadian sleep-wake disorders — before and during their sleep periods (at home).
Genetic and molecular biomarkers	Analysis of biological samples to detect biomarkers that may help in understanding the causes of these circadian rhythm sleep-wake disorders, paving the way for targeted treatments.

Treatment Development	How It Works
Brief flashes (a millisecond) of light in certain wavelengths	Brief flashes of light delivered through goggles and other devices under development enable patients to synchronize the sleep-wake cycle without applying bright light in a continuous manner and avoiding cumbersome light boxes.
Gene editing (for example, CRISPR-Cas9)	This technique edits clock genes that may be mutations or variations that disrupt normal circadian rhythms, which potentially offers a personalized and targeted treatment.
Optogenetics (a technique that uses light to control cells within living tissue)	Invented by Dr. Karl Deisseroth, a researcher at Stanford University, the technique may be applied to adjust circadian rhythms with the goal of precisely controlling the activity of neurons involved in regulating the circadian clock.
Chronobiotics (substances that can shift the timing of circadian rhythms)	Through synthetic biology, the goal is to create new molecules or modify existing ones to enhance effectiveness and specificity in modulating circadian rhythms.

REMEMBER

Advanced chronobiotics, optogenetics, and gene editing could all offer highly targeted, customizable treatments for circadian rhythm disorders. These treatments have the potential for fewer side effects and greater efficacy when compared to traditional pharmacological treatments.

TABLE 12-4 **Parasomnia Disorders**

Diagnosis Technology	How It Works
Portable in-home sleep study devices	Capture parasomnia episodes on a recording device in a natural environment (rather than in a sleep lab situation where proper, comfortable sleep may be difficult).
Synchronized miniature video cameras	Capture parasomnia episodes in a home environment and synch to devices that verify their occurrences during sleep and specific sleep stages.
Treatment Development	**How It Works**
Sound or voice stimuli to abort parasomnia episodes	For patients with NREM and REM parasomnias, a device detects movement and activates a recorded familiar voice (typically a bed partner) that instructs the patient in a soothing tone to relax and subsequently aborts the episode.

Researchers have effectively used the recorded voice approach for treating para-somnias to abort episodes of REM sleep behavior disorder, and the treatment also shows promise for individuals who sleepwalk, particularly children and adolescents.

TABLE 12-5   ## Hypersomnia Disorders

Diagnosis	
Technology	**How It Works**
Apps that measure reaction time	In the testing phase, these apps are designed to measure reaction time to detect daytime sleepiness and potentially may help in the detection of hypersomnia disorders.
Treatment	
Development	**How It Works**
Medications in the pipeline to treat hypersomnia	Treats symptoms of hypersomnia by various methods, for example, helping to consolidate sleep, maintain alertness, or reducing excessive daytime sleepiness, primarily by acting on neurotransmitters in the brain.
Orexin agonists (drugs that mimic the action of the brain chemical orexin)	Further investigations into drugs that target orexin receptors in the brain to address the loss of the orexin peptide (which promotes wakefulness).
Smart polytherapy	Uses multiple drugs — that target different wakefulness pathways — in combination with the goal of optimizing symptom control and minimizing side effects.

Several medications for the treatment of narcolepsy exist, but currently you find only one FDA-approved medication for the treatment of idiopathic hypersomnia. However, this situation will undoubtedly change in the near future, given the increase in studies exploring new medications to treat narcolepsy and other hypersomnias.

TABLE 12-6   ## Insomnia Disorders

Diagnosis	
Technology	**How It Works**
Apps (including Sleep Reset, SleepWatch, Pillow, Sleep Cycle, PrimeNap, and Somryst)	Helps you track nightly sleep patterns and track circadian rhythms that can inform an insomnia diagnosis.
Wearables	Incorporates (in future devices) more advanced biometric sensors to monitor not only sleep stages, but also neurological and physiological responses for deeper insights into causes of insomnia.

Treatment Development	How It Works
IoT (Internet of Things) integration	Provides connections between sleep apps and smart home devices to create an optimal sleep environment by, for example, adjusting bedroom lighting, temperature, and sound based on your sleep cycle and preferences.
App personalization	Uses data from sources such as daily activities, diet, and mental health status to provide a holistic approach that has comprehensive insights and customized sleep recommendations for managing insomnia.
Digital CBT-I	Addresses cognitive behavioral therapy for insomnia with digital therapeutic apps that involve patient input regarding sleep and sleep schedule. The input is tracked over time and used to provide interventions and instructions to help improve sleep.
Orexin antagonists (sleeping pills under development)	Blocks orexin receptors and thereby helps promote sleep for those with insomnia.

REMEMBER

Although digital CBT-I can be highly effective for treating insomnia, in-person CBT-I relies on the input of psychologists specializing in behavioral sleep medicine during face-to-face sessions. These in-person sessions with a psychologist are still the gold standard for treating insomnia.

Finding Additional Support

As the landscape of sleep health evolves, the future of support for individuals with sleep disorders is set to become more dynamic and inclusive. Emerging trends indicate that support groups, social media, and online communities will play increasingly significant roles in providing assistance and fostering connections among those affected by sleep disorders.

Support groups and peer networks

Looking ahead to the future of traditional support groups, expect them to expand in-person and online. Organizations like the Narcolepsy Network already facilitate national online peer-led support group meetings via virtual platforms like Zoom, which ensures that you can access support, regardless of your location. As technology advances, these virtual support groups will become more sophisticated, potentially incorporating interactive tools and resources to enhance engagement and support.

Social media and online communities

Social media platforms and online communities are also transforming how you can find support and resources for sleep disorders. Dedicated groups on Facebook, X (formerly Twitter), and specialized forums provide instant access to a wealth of information and peer support. These platforms enable you to connect with others, share your journey, and access the latest research and treatment options.

REMEMBER

As time goes on, your physical location will continue to be less of an obstacle to receiving care for sleep disorders. The rise of telehealth and virtual consultations — which dramatically increased since the start of the COVID-19 pandemic (declared worldwide in March of 2020) — continues to offer the convenience of receiving professional advice and connecting with experts from the comfort of your home.

Whether through in-person groups, online forums, or innovative digital tools, look for these emerging trends to enhance your ability to achieve better sleep health and overall well-being.

5

The Part of Tens

Find out about conditions and situations that can keep you from a good night's sleep.

Learn how frequent difficulty falling or staying asleep, gasping for air at night, unusual sleep-related movements or behavior, or feeling unrefreshed in the morning might indicate you need professional help.

Chapter **13**

Ten Problems That Can Prevent Restful Sleep

We've all had nights where sleep feels impossible, but for many, struggling to get enough rest is a chronic issue. Whether you have trouble falling asleep, staying asleep, or waking up feeling rested, the barriers between you and a good night's sleep might be more common than you think. Sleep is essential for maintaining physical health, mental well-being, and even emotional balance, but so many factors — ranging from minor annoyances to serious medical issues — can disrupt precious sleep.

This chapter looks at the top ten challenges that could be robbing you of the sleep your body craves. From noisy neighbors and restless pets to underlying medical conditions and anxiety, you can not only explore the causes but also glean actionable solutions to tackle each problem. By identifying and addressing common sleep blockers, you can make informed decisions to protect your sleep and improve your overall quality of life.

A Medical Condition

Medical issues such as chronic pain, heart disease, or asthma can wreak havoc on your sleep. For instance, pain from conditions like arthritis might flare up at night, making it hard for you to fall or stay asleep. Ignoring medical conditions can lead to long-term sleep deprivation, which only worsens your overall health. Treating the root of the problem (the medical condition) is essential for both better sleep and improved well-being.

Common medical conditions that affect sleep include

>> **Asthma:** Breathing difficulties, especially at night, can cause frequent awakenings and prevent deep, restful sleep.

>> **Chronic obstructive pulmonary disease (COPD):** Breathing difficulties may worsen at night, leading to restless sleep and awakenings.

>> **Chronic pain (stemming from arthritis or fibromyalgia, for example):** Pain flare-ups can make finding a comfortable sleep position difficult and contribute to frequent awakenings and struggles to fall asleep.

>> **Diabetes:** Frequent urination due to high blood sugar levels can cause nighttime awakenings, disrupting sleep cycles.

>> **Enlarged prostate:** Nighttime awakenings due to an urge to urinate can also result in fragmented sleep.

>> **Gastroesophageal reflux disease (GERD):** Lying down can exacerbate acid reflux, leading to heartburn and discomfort that interrupts sleep.

>> **Heart disease (such as heart failure):** Breathing problems and discomfort from fluid buildup in the lungs or extremities can lead to poor sleep quality and frequent waking.

>> **Hyperthyroidism:** An overactive thyroid can cause symptoms such as an increased heart rate and anxiety, which can, in turn, cause difficulty with falling and staying asleep.

>> **Kidney disease:** Toxins in the blood due to impaired kidney function can disrupt sleep and cause symptoms similar to those of restless leg syndrome (see Chapter 8). These symptoms can keep you from getting into a comfortable position for sleep.

>> **Menopause:** Hormonal changes — particularly those characterized by hot flashes and night sweats — may result in frequent disruptions in sleep and difficulty staying asleep.

>> **Parkinson's disease:** Tremors, stiffness, and difficulty turning in bed can make sleeping comfortably hard to do. This situation can lead to fragmented sleep.

>> **Skin conditions:** Eczema and psoriasis, for example, can cause itching and discomfort that may make it difficult to fall asleep (and fall back asleep if you awaken).

TIP

If you're dealing with a known medical issue, talk to your doctor about how it might be affecting your sleep. In some cases, adjusting medications, changing your sleep position, or managing symptoms with specialized treatments can make a big difference. For example, people with acid reflux might benefit from raising the head of their bed, while those with chronic pain could look into body pillows for extra support.

A Sleep Disorder

Sleep disorders are much more common than many people realize, and they can have a significant impact on your sleep quality. Insomnia, restless legs syndrome (RLS), and obstructive sleep apnea (OSA) are just a few examples of sleep disorders that might be keeping you up at night.

>> **Insomnia,** the most common sleep disorder, can make falling or staying asleep difficult. This disorder often results in waking up feeling unrefreshed.

>> **RLS** causes an irresistible urge to move your legs that you can relieve only by doing so. Experiencing this syndrome can keep you awake for hours.

>> **OSA,** a condition in which breathing repeatedly stops and starts during sleep, often goes undiagnosed because people don't realize it's happening. Many times they seek help only after years of always feeling sleepy.

For more details on various sleep disorders, including insomnia, RLS, and OSA, see Chapters 7 and 8. If you suspect that you have a sleep disorder, don't hesitate to see a specialist (turn to Chapter 9 for more on how to find one). Participating in a sleep study (also in Chapter 9) can help diagnose these issues, and treatment options range from medications to devices like CPAP machines for those with OSA.

WARNING

If you don't seek treatment for your sleep disorders, you may experience serious health complications as a result. These conditions may include heart disease, diabetes, and depression.

Your Bedpartner

Sharing a bed can be comforting, but your partner's sleep habits can be more disruptive than you realize. Whether you experience their snoring, frequent movements, or the age-old battle for blankets, your bedpartner may be preventing you from achieving deep, restful sleep.

Even seemingly small things, such as your partner's phone screen lighting up in the middle of the night, can disturb your sleep cycle. And if your partner has a sleep disorder — for example, sleep apnea — their tossing and turning can be a major source of disruption for you as well.

TIP

Communicate with your partner about the impact their sleep habits have on your rest. You might need to get creative with solutions if your bedpartner has continued restlessness during sleep. You can

>> Trade one larger bed for two smaller beds by moving twin beds together. This solution can minimize mattress movement that might be disturbing your sleep.

>> Use separate blankets to avoid the blanket battle.

>> Wear a sleep mask to block out the phone screen's light.

For more serious issues like snoring, your partner may benefit from medical treatment or lifestyle changes, such as losing weight, avoiding alcohol, or using nasal strips.

REMEMBER

Your sleep matters just as much as your bedpartner's does. If sharing a bed consistently disrupts your sleep, you may even want to consider sleeping in separate rooms occasionally (colloquially known as a *sleep divorce*) to ensure that both of you get the rest you need to stay healthy and happy.

Co-Sleeping with Your Children

Although some parents swear by the closeness brought on by co-sleeping (sharing a bed) with their children, others struggle with the lack of space, constant movement, and inevitable disruptions to their sleep. Children often shift positions, kick, or wake up seeking parental comfort throughout the night.

WARNING

For parents of newborns or toddlers, co-sleeping might feel like the easiest way to manage midnight wake-ups. But this solution can quickly become a habit that affects your ability to get restful sleep. And without enough rest, you may find yourself more irritable, less focused, and less able to keep up with your day-to-day parenting (and other) tasks. In addition, the American Academy of Pediatrics Task Force on Sudden Infant Death Syndrome (SIDS) and the Committee on the Fetus and Newborn recommends that infants sleep in the parents' room, close to the parents' bed, but on a separate surface designed for infants. This sleeping situation should ideally last for at least the first six months due to the potential risk of SIDS from co-sleeping.

If co-sleeping is affecting your rest, set boundaries for when and where it happens. Consider transitioning your child to their own room, or use a co-sleeping crib that attaches to your bed but still provides some separation. Another option involves allowing your children (except for newborns) to sleep with you only during naps, which keeps nighttime for sleeping by yourself.

Dogs, Cats, and Other Pets

Although many people find comfort in having their pets close by, it's important to assess whether sleeping with your pet compromises your sleep quality. Pets are beloved members of the family, but sharing your bed with them can seriously disrupt your sleep. Animals can be more active at night, and they tend to shift positions, wake up to scratch or clean themselves, and even demand attention at odd hours. Allergies to pet dander can also cause nasal congestion and sneezing, making it hard to breathe comfortably.

REMEMBER

Optimize your sleep setup for your own comfort, not your pet's. Prioritizing your sleep doesn't mean you love them any less — it just means you need to set healthy limits.

TIP

Create a cozy sleeping space for your pets outside of your bed. Train them to sleep in their own beds, either on the floor or in a separate room, if necessary. If they must sleep in the room with you, consider using pet gates to establish boundaries.

Noise and Light

Even small amounts of noise or light can prevent you from getting deep, restful sleep. Although you may think that you've adapted to the street sounds outside your window or the hum of the fan, these noises can still interfere with your ability to stay asleep. Similarly, even the glow from your phone or an alarm clock can disrupt your natural sleep-wake cycle by signaling to your brain that it's not fully dark, which interferes with melatonin production. To read more on environmental factors and external disturbances to sleep, check out Chapter 3.

Invest in blackout curtains or a sleep mask to block out light, and consider using earplugs or a white noise machine to drown out disruptive sounds. Try to cut out screen time (even if using blue-blocking apps) at least 30 minutes before bed, and move any electronics away from your bed because they emit low levels of light even when turned off.

Mattresses and Pillows

If you've been waking up with a sore back or neck, or you find yourself tossing and turning, your mattress or pillow might be to blame. A mattress that's too soft or too firm can leave you uncomfortable, and an old or unsupportive pillow can strain your neck. Both situations can lead to disrupted sleep.

Your sleep position also plays a role in determining the best mattress and pillow for you. Side sleepers, for instance, need more cushioning for their hips and shoulders, while back sleepers may benefit from firmer support.

Replace your mattress every seven to ten years, or sooner if it's showing signs of wear such as sagging or lumps. As you age, the discomfort from poor mattresses or pillows can have a significant effect on your sleep quality, especially if you have joint or back pain. Choose a pillow based on your preferred sleep position — side sleepers generally need thicker pillows. Your pillow should support your head and neck but not reach under your shoulders.

Investing in a good mattress and pillow is an investment in your health. Don't skimp on these sleep essentials; you spend a third of your life in bed!

Worries, Anxiety, or Depression

Falling asleep may feel impossible when your mind is racing with thoughts about the day, worries about the future, or feelings of sadness. Anxiety and depression are two of the most common mental health issues that can wreak havoc on your sleep. Anxiety tends to make falling asleep trickier, and depression can cause both insomnia and oversleeping.

In the middle of the night, worries often seem magnified, and you may have trouble getting back to sleep after you awaken. If you don't seek treatment, your mental health challenges can lead to a vicious cycle of poor sleep, which can then exacerbate anxiety or depression.

For a deep dive into the relationship between sleep and mental health, refer to Chapter 3. If your worries, anxiety, or depression are seriously affecting your sleep, seek professional help. Cognitive behavioral therapy for insomnia (CBT-I) has been shown to be highly effective in treating sleep disturbances related to mental health issues.

Incorporate relaxation techniques into your bedtime routine to help calm your mind. Practices such as deep breathing, progressive muscle relaxation, or mindfulness meditation can be particularly helpful. Journaling before bed is another way to clear your mind of lingering thoughts.

Your Bedtime Routine (or Lack Thereof)

Your bedtime routine sets the stage for a good night's sleep. If you don't have a consistent routine, your body might not be ready to sleep when your head hits the pillow. And even worse, having inconsistent bedtimes can confuse your internal clock and make falling asleep or waking up feeling rested harder. Your wake-up time has the most impact on keeping your sleep-wake rhythm in place, so even if you go to bed later than usual, keep your wake-up time the same.

Many people struggle with winding down, especially in our tech-heavy world where screens and distractions are everywhere. It's easy to fall into the trap of scrolling through your phone right up until bedtime, but this habit can leave your brain too stimulated to fall asleep.

Establish a consistent pre-bedtime routine that helps signal to your body it's time to wind down. Assuming these activities help you fall asleep, you can try incorporating reading from a physical book — not a screen — and make sure that your reading light is just bright enough to be able to discern the words on the page. You can also listen to calming music, try meditation, or take a warm bath. Stick to your bedtime routine as much as possible, even on weekends. A consistent schedule helps regulate your body's internal clock so that falling asleep and waking up at the right times happen as they should.

Here's an example of a beneficial bedtime routine for adults, broken down by time:

>> **1 hour before bed:** Turn off electronic devices. Shut down your phone, tablet, and TV to reduce exposure to blue light, which can interfere with melatonin production and make falling asleep more difficult. Dim the lights. Lowering the brightness in your environment signals to your body that it's time to wind down.

>> **45 minutes before bed:** Journal or write a to-do list. If you tend to worry about tasks for the next day, jot them down to clear your mind. This can help prevent the anxiety of looming tasks from keeping you awake. Practice mindfulness or meditation: Spend a few minutes practicing mindfulness or deep breathing exercises to quiet your mind and reduce stress.

>> **30 minutes before bed:** Take a warm bath or shower. A warm bath helps relax your muscles, and as your body cools down afterward, it signals to your brain that it's time for sleep.

>> **15 minutes before bed:** Engage in a relaxing activity. Try reading a book, doing some light stretching, or practicing deep breathing exercises. Avoid stimulating activities like work or intense discussions.

>> **5 minutes before bed:** Brush teeth and complete any last-minute personal hygiene tasks to signal to your body that you're preparing for sleep.

>> **Right at bedtime:** Get into bed. Make sure that your bedroom is cool, dark, and quiet. Use earplugs or a white noise machine if necessary. Focus on relaxing thoughts: After you're in bed, think about calming or positive thoughts, or try a guided visualization to help you drift off to sleep. Bring your attention to your breathing and follow it with your mind.

Sleep Habits

Your sleep habits go beyond just what you do right before bed (see the preceding section). How much caffeine you consume, whether you exercise during the day, and even how much natural sunlight you get can all influence your sleep quality. Napping for too long during the day, eating heavy meals, or consuming alcohol right before bed can also disrupt your sleep. To learn more about how diet, exercise, and other habits affect your sleep, journey over to Chapter 6.

A regular sleep schedule is one of the most important habits to develop because it helps regulate your body's circadian rhythm (see Chapter 4). When you go to bed and wake up at the same time every day, your body becomes more efficient at falling and staying asleep.

TIP

Set a sleep schedule and stick to it. Try to go to bed and wake up at the same time every day, even on weekends. Additionally, limit caffeine intake after noon, avoid heavy meals close to bedtime, and aim for at least 30 minutes of exercise daily to promote better sleep.

Chapter **14**

Ten Signs That You Should See a Sleep Specialist

Maybe you've had one too many nights lying awake, counting sheep while the clock ticks on. Or perhaps you're nodding off in the middle of meetings, feeling like coffee is the only thing keeping you upright. Sleep can be elusive, and when problems with getting sufficient sleep begin piling up, you may wonder whether something more serious is going on. While an occasional sleepless night or mid-afternoon yawn is normal, persistent sleep troubles might indicate an underlying issue that only a specialist can help address.

This chapter dives into the top ten signs that you might need to call in a pro — someone who can decode what's going on with your sleep situation and help you finally get the rest you need. Sleep issues are incredibly common, and you're not alone. Many people struggle with sleep issues — whether temporary or long-term — and you don't need to feel embarrassed or discouraged.

Taking steps to improve your sleep is an act of self-care, and reaching out for help when you need it is a positive, proactive choice. Sleep specialists have a wide range of tools and treatments to help you regain restful nights. Sometimes a single consultation can give you the answers and peace of mind you need!

You're Not Able to Fall Asleep

Occasional difficulty falling asleep is normal, but if lying awake at night has become a regular pattern for you, you might be struggling with a sleep disorder. You may find yourself lying in bed for hours, unable to stop racing thoughts or find a comfortable position.

If you're spending more than 30 minutes trying to fall asleep at least three times a week, or if you have struggled with sleeplessness for more than a month, it's a good idea to consult a sleep specialist (see Chapter 9).

Persistent difficulty falling asleep could stem from

>> **Insomnia:** Persistent sleeplessness, often initially triggered stress or anxiety, can make falling asleep feel like a battle.

>> **Circadian rhythm sleep-wake disruptions:** Misalignment in your body's internal clock, particularly a delayed sleep-wake phase disorder, can make falling asleep at the desired time hard to do.

>> **Restless legs syndrome (RLS):** An urge to move your legs — that is worse at bedtime and at rest but is temporarily relieved by leg movement — can result in difficulty falling asleep.

WARNING

Each of these disorders may worsen without intervention, and ignoring them can make a short-term or transient issue into a more chronic condition. Over time, prolonged sleeplessness can lead to frustration and even anxiety surrounding bedtime, creating a cycle that only makes it harder to relax.

You Have Restless or Frequently Disturbed Sleep

If you're waking up three or more times per night, at least three nights per week, your body misses out on critical restorative sleep stages, particularly deep sleep and REM sleep (see Chapter 2 for more about sleep stages). During deep sleep, your body repairs tissues, strengthens the immune system, and releases growth hormones that aid muscle recovery and overall health.

Missing these important sleep stages can leave you feeling physically drained, sore, or more susceptible to illness. Restless sleep can stem from conditions such as sleep apnea, periodic limb movement disorder (PLMD), or even environmental issues like light or noise in your bedroom. Over time, restless sleep can lead to a buildup of sleepiness that's hard to shake. To assess whether your restlessness might be concerning, consider the following:

>> **Duration:** Have your sleep disturbances persisted for over a month?

>> **Frequency:** Are you waking up multiple times each night, at least three nights per week?

>> **Impact:** Do you often wake up feeling sleepy, tired, moody, or foggy?

If you answered "yes" to one or more of these questions, a sleep specialist can help uncover what's keeping you from experiencing truly restful sleep and find solutions to help you stay asleep through the night.

You Wake up Gasping, Gagging, or Choking During Your Sleep

Waking up gasping for air or feeling like you're choking can be alarming and may indicate a sleep-related breathing disorder. If you wake up gasping or choking multiple times a week, or if you experience this with loud snoring, morning head-aches, or a dry mouth, it's time to consult a specialist. These signs often indicate a treatable condition that, after medical attention, can greatly improve your sleep and well-being.

People who experience these episodes could also have

>> **Obstructive sleep apnea (OSA),** where the muscles in your upper airway relax too much and block the passage of air to your lungs.

>> **Gastroesophageal reflux disease (GERD),** which can cause stomach acid to rise into your throat at night, creating a choking sensation.

>> **Nocturnal asthma,** a situation in which asthma symptoms can worsen during sleep, leading to breathing difficulties.

Sudden wake-ups not only disturb your sleep cycle but may also increase your risk for other health issues if you don't address them. Persistent episodes of unpleasant awakenings can contribute to daytime sleepiness, headaches, and elevated blood pressure.

You Consistently Feel Unrefreshed in the Morning

If you regularly feel groggy in the morning or throughout the day, despite getting seven to eight hours of sleep, you may not be getting the restorative rest your body needs. Similarly, if daytime sleepiness or fatigue affects your mood, memory, focus, or quality of life, seeing a sleep specialist may be what you need. Consistently feeling unrefreshed isn't something you have to just live with.

Emotionally, poor-quality sleep can heighten irritability and moodiness, lower your tolerance for stress, and increase feelings of anxiety or sadness. When your mind and body aren't fully recharged, even minor challenges can feel overwhelming. You may find yourself making more mistakes, struggling with motivation, or needing extra time to complete tasks.

Without restorative sleep, you may experience grogginess, mood swings, and cognitive issues. And you may not even realize that you aren't experiencing full alertness. Over time, sleep that doesn't leave you feeling rested can take a toll on both your productivity and your emotional well-being. Without restorative sleep, your brain has a harder time concentrating, solving problems, and processing information, which can make staying organized and efficient during the day difficult to do.

Common culprits that can cause a lack of refreshing sleep include

>> **Circadian rhythm sleep-wake disorders:** Misaligned sleep schedules can interfere with the quality of your sleep.

>> **Insomnia:** Difficulty falling or staying asleep can result in shortened sleep or fragmented sleep cycles, respectively, leaving you unrefreshed.

>> **Sleep apnea:** Frequent breathing interruptions prevent your body from reaching deep sleep stages.

You can find these sleep disorders and others covered in Chapters 7 and 8.

You Have Significant Difficulty Staying Awake During the Day

Daytime drowsiness is normal after an occasional poor night's sleep, but if you're struggling to stay awake most days, an underlying issue may be responsible. If you nod off unintentionally, or have experienced this pattern for more than a month, seeing a specialist is a good idea. Excessive daytime sleepiness — especially if it affects safety or focus — is a strong indicator of a sleep disorder.

Persistent daytime drowsiness is often linked to

>> **Chronic insomnia:** Poor-quality sleep leads to reduced alertness and energy during the day.

>> **Circadian rhythm sleep-wake misalignment:** If your circadian rhythms aren't in synch with your work life, you can be drowsy when you need to be awake.

>> **Idiopathic hypersomnia:** This refers to daytime sleepiness of unclear causes.

>> **Medical conditions:** Pain, frequent urination, and heart conditions can result in delayed or interrupted sleep leading to daytime sleepiness.

>> **Narcolepsy:** This neurological condition causes sudden, overwhelming episodes of sleepiness that are known as *sleep attacks*.

>> **Sleep apnea:** Repeated interruptions throughout the night can lead to significant daytime sleepiness and fatigue.

WARNING

Falling asleep unexpectedly — especially during critical activities such as driving — can put your safety at risk and significantly impact daily functioning.

You Have Attention, Memory, or Mood Problems Along with Daytime Fatigue or Sleepiness

Sleep is crucial for cognitive functions and emotional balance, so the fact that poor sleep can make you irritable, forgetful, or unfocused is no surprise. If you're frequently experiencing brain fog, memory lapses, or mood swings, you may be experiencing sleep disruptions caused by disorders such as sleep apnea, insomnia, periodic limb movements, an irregular sleep schedule, or circadian rhythm misalignment (delayed or advanced sleep-wake phases).

To determine if your cognitive and mood issues could be sleep-related, ask yourself about these factors:

>> **Frequency:** Are mood swings, focus problems, or memory lapses occurring multiple times per week?

>> **Pattern:** Has this pattern of issues lasted more than a few weeks?

>> **Sleepiness:** Do these issues coincide with feelings of daytime sleepiness or fatigue?

If these patterns sound familiar, a specialist can help evaluate whether your mental clarity or emotional stability is being affected by poor sleep —whether the cause is insufficient sleep duration or quality. With improved sleep, these symptoms may disappear or at least become easier to manage.

You Snore and/or Have Breathing Pauses While You Sleep

Snoring — especially loud, disruptive snoring — paired with breathing pauses may be more than just an annoyance to your bed partner. It can be a sign of obstructive sleep apnea (OSA), a condition in which your upper airway becomes partially or fully blocked during sleep. These blockages reduce oxygen levels, disrupt sleep cycles, and can leave you feeling drowsy during the day. And you may not even be aware of waking up multiple times throughout the night.

If you've been told that you snore loudly most nights or that you sometimes stop breathing during sleep, you should consider having a sleep evaluation (see Chapter 9). Consulting a sleep specialist can help clarify what's behind these symptoms. A professional can assess whether OSA or another condition is affecting your sleep and recommend treatments — such as CPAP therapy, oral appliances, upper airway surgery, or lifestyle adjustments — that could make a huge difference for both you and your bedpartner.

Additionally, here are some other signs to watch for:

>> **Excessive daytime sleepiness:** Feeling tired, groggy, or unfocused throughout the day, even after what seems like a full night's sleep.

>> **Morning headaches:** A telltale sign of poor oxygen flow during the night.

>> **Night sweats:** Can be a symptom of medical conditions or simply a sleeping environment that is too warm, but night sweats can also be associated with OSA.

>> **Sore throat:** Waking up with a dry, scratchy, or sore throat can indicate snoring-related airway irritation.

WARNING

Ignoring loud snoring and breathing pauses isn't just annoying for those around you — it can also increase health risks. Left untreated, conditions such as OSA can lead to high blood pressure, heart disease, cardiac arrhythmias, and increased daytime sleepiness or fatigue, impacting your overall quality of life.

Your Bedpartner Describes Unusual Behaviors During Your Sleep

If your bed partner has noticed that you're talking, moving, or even acting out dreams while asleep, you may be dealing with a parasomnia — a group of sleep disorders that includes conditions like REM sleep behavior disorder (RBD), sleep-walking, or sleep (night) terrors. These behaviors can range from harmless mumbling to complex movements or actions. You might not be aware of these episodes, but they can disrupt your bed partner's sleep, create unease, or even pose safety risks if physical movements are involved. See Chapter 8 for more information on these types of disorders.

TIP

If you live alone and suspect you're experiencing unusual sleep behaviors, consider setting up a simple audio-video recording to capture what's happening at night.

To determine if your sleep behaviors warrant professional help, consider these factors:

>> **Frequency:** Are these actions occurring at least once or twice a month? An occasional episode may not be a concern, but frequent incidents could indicate a deeper issue.

>> **Disruption:** Are these actions disturbing you or your bed partner's sleep by vocalizations or body movements?

>> **Impact:** Do these behaviors involve risky actions such as getting out of bed, moving around, or interacting with objects? Such behaviors (for example, bumping into furniture, knocking things over, opening doors or windows, and striking out or kicking) can lead to potential safety risks for you and your bed partner.

WARNING

If these sleep behaviors are frequent, disruptive, or affect your safety or that of others, don't brush them off. Left unaddressed, some parasomnias can escalate and pose greater risks over time.

You Have an Involuntary Urge to Move Your Limbs at Bedtime

If you feel an uncontrollable urge to move your legs, especially at night, it may be due to restless legs syndrome (RLS). RLS can cause uncomfortable sensations, such as tingling, itching, or a creepy-crawly feeling that prompts you to shift or move your legs. This situation often disrupts your ability to relax and drift off to sleep because you feel that you must move your legs. As a result, you can fail to get a good night's rest. Over time, this lack of restful sleep can lead to persistent fatigue, irritability, and even impact your mood or focus during the day.

Consider seeking professional support if you find yourself experiencing this urge most nights, if it's frequent enough to disrupt your sleep, or if you notice that these sensations are

>> **Accompanied by leg movements during sleep:** About 80 percent of those with RLS have periodic limb movements during sleep. These limb movements can fragment sleep and create a vicious cycle: RLS makes falling asleep difficult, and if you wake up from the periodic limb movements, it also makes falling back to sleep difficult.

>> **Persistent:** If these sensations have lasted for over a month and are affecting your sleep quality, it's time to consult a specialist.

>> **Triggered by medications:** Certain medications, such as antihistamines or antidepressants, can worsen symptoms. If you notice this link, bring it up with your doctor.

>> **Worse when you feel stress:** Stress often intensifies RLS symptoms, which makes relaxing at bedtime even harder.

You Habitually Fall Sleep and Wake Up Earlier or Later Than You Desire

If your sleep-wake schedule feels consistently out of sync with your life, you may have a circadian rhythm sleep-wake disorder, such as delayed sleep-wake phase disorder (DSWPD) or advanced sleep-wake phase disorder (ASWPD). You may find that falling asleep or waking up at conventional times is difficult for you. This situation can lead to missed appointments, lateness to work, and difficulty participating in social events.

See a sleep specialist for these symptoms if

» You're regularly struggling to sleep or wake at desired times (at least three times a week).

» This pattern has persisted for at least three months.

» You do go to sleep (earlier or later) and get up (earlier or later) as you wish and your sleep duration and quality improve.

These patterns often indicate a circadian rhythm sleep-wake misalignment that may benefit from light therapy or chronotherapy.

Appendix A

In this appendix, you can find four tables (Tables A-1 through A-4) that offer details about specific areas of the brain involved in sleep, natural chemical substances that have an effect on wakefulness and sleep, and prescription medications (for treating sleep disorders). I cover related content primarily in Chapter 4.

TABLE A-1 **Key Sleep-Wake Brain Areas and Neurotransmitters**

Structure	What It Promotes	Neurotransmitter	Key Facts about the Structure
Reticular formation (RF)	Wake	Glutamate	Comprises the central core of the brainstem and contains major ascending and descending neuronal pathways. Large lesions in this area result in decreased wakefulness and subsequent coma.
Locus coeruleus (LC)	Wake	Norepinephrine	Located in the pons of the brainstem, and receives neuronal input from the VLPO, and output to the cortex. Lesions in this area can reduce wakefulness and enhance sleep.
Raphe nuclei (RN)	Wake	Serotonin	Located in the brainstem, and receives neuronal input from the VLPO, and output to the cortex.
Tuberomammillary nucleus (TMN)	Wake	Histamine	Located in the hypothalamus, and receives neuronal input from the VLPO, and output to the cortex.
Laterodorsal tegmental (LDT) and Pedunculopontine tegmental (PPT) nuclei	Wake REM Sleep	Acetylcholine	Located in the brainstem, and output to the thalamus.
Ventral tegmental area (VTA) and substantia nigra (SN)	Wake	Dopamine	Connects to the forebrain regions that influence emotional and motor behavior.

(continued)

Structure	What It Promotes	Neurotransmitter	Key Facts about the Structure
Basal forebrain (BF)	Wake REM sleep	Acetylcholine Glutamate Gamma-Aminobutyric Acid	Connects to the brainstem and hypothalamus, and stimulates cortical activation during both wakefulness and REM sleep.
Ventrolateral preoptic (VLPO) nucleus	Sleep	Galanin	Located in the hypothalamus; lesions in this area can cause insomnia.
Median preoptic nucleus (MnPN)	Sleep	Gamma-Aminobutyric Acid	Located in the preoptic anterior hypothalamus (POAH) of the preoptic area (POA); lesions in this area cause insomnia.

TABLE A-2   Naturally Occurring Sleep–Wake Substances

Substance	What It Is	Where It Is in the Brain	Sleep-Wake Effect
Acetylcholine	Neurotransmitter	Basal forebrain, brainstem	Promotes both wakefulness and REM sleep
Adenosine	Chemical found in all cells	Basal forebrain	Promotes sleep
Dopamine	Neurotransmitter (excitatory/inhibitory) and hormone	Hypothalamus, substantia nigra (SN), ventral tegmental area (VTA)	Promotes wakefulness
Epinephrine	Neurotransmitter (excitatory) and hormone	Brainstem (medulla)	Promotes wakefulness
Galanin	Neuropeptide (protein-like molecule that is produced and released by neurons; primarily inhibitory)	Primarily hypothalamus	Promotes sleep
Gamma-aminobutyric acid	Neurotransmitter (inhibitory)	Throughout the brain including the brainstem	Promotes sleep

Substance	What It Is	Where It Is in the Brain	Sleep-Wake Effect
Glutamate	Neurotransmitter (excitatory) and amino acid	Throughout the brain	Promotes both sleep and wakefulness
Glycine	Neurotransmitter (inhibitory) and amino acid	Throughout the brain including the brainstem	Promotes sleep
Growth hormone–releasing hormone (GHRH)	Hormone that stimulates the release of growth hormone	Hypothalamus	Promotes sleep
Histamine	Neurotransmitter (excitatory/inhibitory)	Tuberomammillary nucleus (TMN)	Promotes wakefulness and suppresses REM sleep
Interleukin-1β	Cytokine (protein important in cell signaling and immune function; excitatory/inhibitory)	Throughout the brain, but mainly in hippocampus	Promotes sleep (NREM)
Melatonin	Hormone (inhibitory)	Pineal gland	Promotes sleep and inhibits wake-promoting signals
Nitric oxide	Gaseous signaling molecule considered a neurotransmitter (excitatory/inhibitory)	Throughout the brain	Promotes both sleep and wakefulness
Norepinephrine	Neurotransmitter (excitatory/inhibitory) and hormone	Locus coeruleus (LC)	Promotes wakefulness
Orexin (hypocretin)	Neurotransmitter (excitatory/inhibitory)	Primarily hypothalamus	Regulates sleep and wakefulness
Prostaglandin-D2	Prostaglandin (hormone-like substances that affect several body functions, such as pain/inflammation; excitatory/inhibitory)	Throughout the brain	Promotes sleep
Serotonin	Neurotransmitter (inhibitory)	Primarily raphe nuclei	Promotes both sleep and wakefulness
Tumor necrosis factor-α	Cytokine	Throughout the brain	Promotes sleep

TABLE A-3   FDA-Approved Prescription Sleeping Pills for Insomnia

Compound	Class	How it works
Daridorexant	Dual orexin receptor antagonist (DORA)	Binds to both orexin receptors OX1 and OX2 to block the wake-promotion effects of orexins A and B
Diazepam	Benzodiazepine	Binds to $GABA_A$ receptors to increase GABA activity in promoting sleep
Doxepin	Tricyclic antidepressant	Primarily binds to histamine (H_1) receptors to block its wake-promoting effects
Estazolam	Benzodiazepine	Binds to $GABA_A$ receptors to increase GABA activity in promoting sleep
Eszopiclone	Non-benzodiazepine	Binds to $GABA_A$ receptors to increase GABA activity in promoting sleep
Flurazepam	Benzodiazepine	Binds to $GABA_A$ receptors to increase GABA activity in promoting sleep
Lemborexant	Dual orexin receptor antagonist (DORA)	Binds to both orexin receptors OXR1 and OXR2 to block the wake-promotion effects of orexins A and B
Lorazepam	Benzodiazepine	Binds to $GABA_A$ receptors to increase GABA activity in promoting sleep
Quazepam	Benzodiazepine	Binds to $GABA_A$ receptors to increase GABA activity in promoting sleep
Ramelteon	Melatonin receptor agonist	Mimics melatonin sleep-promoting and circadian effects by binding to melatonin MT_1 and MT_2 receptors in the suprachiasmatic nucleus (SCN)
Suvorexant	Dual orexin receptor antagonist (DORA)	Binds to both orexin receptors OXR1 and OXR2 to block the wake-promotion effects of orexins A and B
Temazepam	Benzodiazepine	Binds to $GABA_A$ receptors to increase GABA activity in promoting sleep
Triazolam	Benzodiazepine	Binds to $GABA_A$ receptors to increase GABA activity in promoting sleep
Zaleplon	Non-benzodiazepine	Binds to $GABA_A$ receptors to increase GABA activity in promoting sleep
Zolpidem	Non-benzodiazepine	Binds to $GABA_A$ receptors to increase GABA activity in promoting sleep

TABLE A-4 FDA-Approved Prescription Wake-Promoting/ Stimulant Compounds

Compound	Class	Indications	How it works
Amphetamine	Stimulant	EDS/narcolepsy	Increases dopamine and norepinephrine by boosting secretion and blocking their reuptake in neurons
Armodafinil	Non-amphetamine wake-promoting compound	EDS/narcolepsy, OSA, and shift-work sleep disorder	Primarily blocks dopamine reuptake in neurons to increase brain dopamine levels
Methylphenidate	Stimulant	narcolepsy	Increases dopamine and norepinephrine by boosting secretion and blocking their reuptake in neurons
Modafinil	Non-amphetamine wake-promoting compound	EDS/narcolepsy, OSA, and shift-work sleep disorder	Primarily blocks dopamine reuptake in neurons to increase brain dopamine levels
Pitolisant	Histamine H3 inverse agonist/ antagonist	EDS and cataplexy/ narcolepsy	Primarily blocks histamine receptors to increase brain histamine levels
Sodium oxybate	$GABA_B$ agonist	EDS and cataplexy/ narcolepsy; mixed salts sodium oxybate: EDS/ idiopathic hypersomnia	Primarily bind to $GABA_B$ receptors, which enhances the inhibitory effects of GABA and promotes sleep; low-sodium, once-nightly, and twice nightly medications available
Solriamfetol	Non-amphetamine wake-promoting compound	EDS/OSA and narcolepsy	Blocks dopamine and norepinephrine reuptake in neurons to increase their levels in the brain

Appendix B

This appendix shows a series of actual brain activity measurements for various stages of sleep; the recordings were taken during in-clinic sleep studies by PSG. And you can also find recordings that show the brain activity related to certain sleep disorders.

Brain wave activity during the wake state

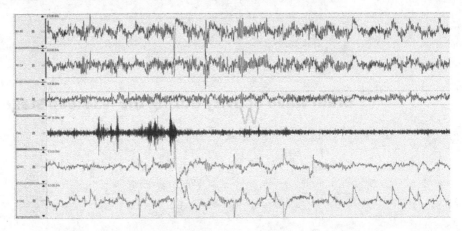

Brain wave activity during the N1 sleep stage

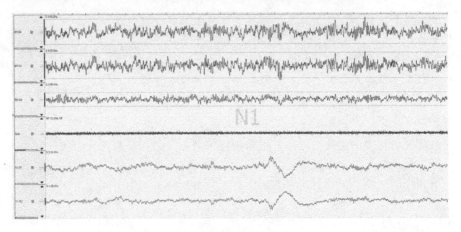

Brain wave activity during the N2 sleep stage

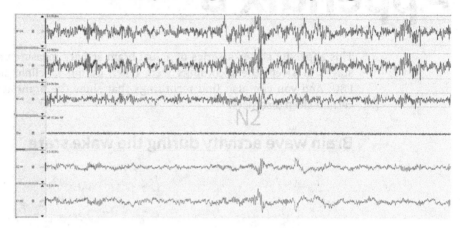

Brain wave activity during the N3 sleep stage

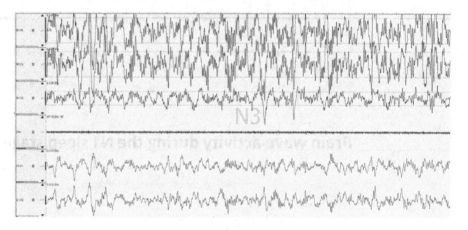

Brain wave activity during the REM sleep state/stage

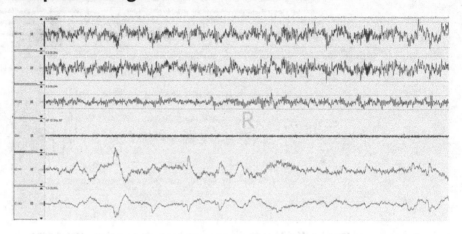

Hypopnea in obstructive sleep apnea

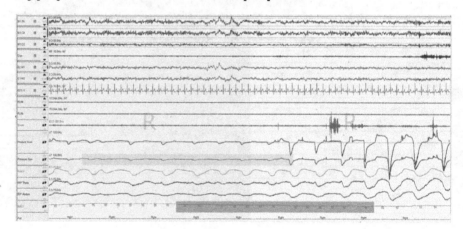

Apnea in obstructive sleep apnea

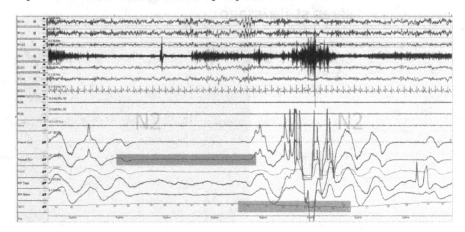

Periodic limb movement disorder (PLMD)

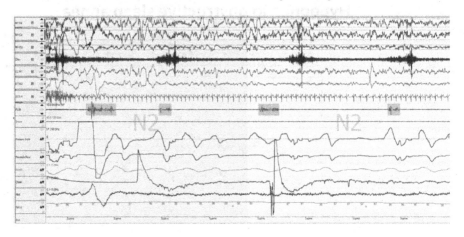

REM sleep behavior disorder

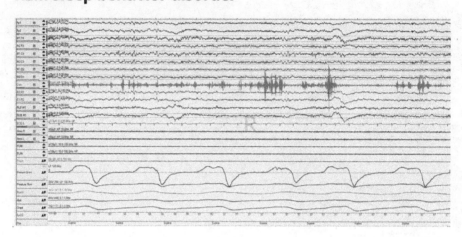

Index

ballistocardiography (BCG), 241

basal forebrain, 86–87, 282

BCG (ballistocardiography), 241

bed-sharing, 127

bedtime routines, 13–15, 233, 267–268

bed-wetting, 186

behavioral consequences, 65–70

behavioral modification therapy (BMT), 177

behavioral sleep medicine psychologist, 204

behavioral therapies, 25, 150

benign sleep myoclonus of infancy, 183

benzodiazepines, 72, 83, 181, 284

beta blockers, 55–56, 115

beta waves, 28, 217

bilevel positive airway pressure (BPAP), 175, 230

biomarker, 104, 254

biphasic sleep, 37

black box approach, 244

black population, 126

blood alcohol concentration (BAC), 65

blood pressure
 nervous system and, 78–79
 during REM sleep, 10
 sleep deprivation and, 62, 93

blood sugar, 61

blood tests, 207–208

blood vessels, 62–63, 96

blue light, 89, 139, 245

BMI (body mass index), 171

BMT (behavioral modification therapy), 177

body movements, 11

body position, 234

body temperature
 impact on sleep, 53
 introduction to, 10, 12
 in rats, 35
 during sleep, 96

books, 35–37

Borbély, Alexander (pharmacologist), 98

bowel function, 94

BPAP (bilevel positive airway pressure), 175, 230

brain activity
 dreams and, 103–104
 during N2 and N3 sleep stages, 288
 during REM sleep and sleep apnea, 289
 during sleep, 11, 30
 sleep deprivation and, 49, 56–60
 during wake state and N1 sleep stage, 287

brainstem, 87, 90

brainwaves, 8, 287–291

breathing
 disorders, 167–177
 exercises, 59, 89
 nervous system and, 78–79
 during sleep, 11, 91–92
 tests, 219
 tracking, 241

bright light therapy, 164–165

bruxism, 182, 219

C

caffeine, 55, 61, 71, 85, 133–134

cannabidiol (CBD), 135

cannabis, 133–134

CAP (cyclic alternating pattern), 90

car accidents, 16

carbohydrates, 19, 68, 131

carbon dioxide monitoring, 220

cardiopulmonary coupling (CPC), 242

cardiovascular disease, 21, 52, 62–63, 93, 168

cardiovascular medications, 55–56

cardiovascular system, 92–93

Carvedilol, 56

cataplexy, 85, 154

catathrenia, 168

catch-up sleep, 93

CBD (cannabidiol), 135

CBT-I (cognitive behavioral therapy for insomnia), 25, 60, 150

CCSH (Certified Clinical Sleep Health educators), 203–204

cerebellum, 87

cerebral anemia theory, 41

cerebral cortex, 48

cerebrospinal fluid (CSF) tests, 207–208

Certified Clinical Sleep Health educators (CCSH), 203–204

Certified Respiratory Therapist (CRT), 203–204

characteristics, sleep, 10–12

charley horse, 181–182

chest cuirass, 178

children
 dreams in, 107–108
 musculoskeletal effects in, 64
 nutrition in, 132
 sleep apnea in, 173–174
 sleep habits in, 13, 19, 128
 sleep optimization in, 137–138

chin muscle movements, 31, 218–219

choking, 273–274

cholinergic neurons, 80

chronic exercise, 136

chronic inflammation, 61

chronic obstructive cardiopulmonary disease (COPD), 55, 63, 262

chronic pain, 262

chronic sleep loss, 20, 51–52

chronic sleepiness, 16

chronic volitional sleep restriction, 51. See also chronic sleep loss

chronobiotics, 255

Chung, Frances (professor), 171

circadian rhythms
 advances in, 254–255
 athletes and, 67–68
 chronobiology and, 97–100
 definition of, 10, 77
 effects on the body, 90–97
 environmental factors and, 52–53
 medications and, 82–85
 nervous system and, 78–82
 in nonhumans, 39
 regulating, 85–90

Q

quantified self movement, 244
quazepam, 83, 284
questionnaire, 199
quiet sleep, 34

R

racial differences, 11, 126–127
ramelteon, 83, 151, 284
raphe nuclei (RN), 81, 86, 281
rapid eye movement. *See* REM (rapid eye movement)
RBD (REM sleep behavior disorder), 90, 113, 125, 187–189
RDI (respiratory disturbance index), 234
reactive co-sleeping, 138
rebound insomnia, 83
Rechtschaffen, Allan (professor), 41
recovery, 42
referral, sleep medicine, 196–197
refined sugars, 19, 130
Registered Polysomnographic Technologists (RPSGT), 203
Registered Respiratory Therapist (RRT), 203–204
Registered Sleep Technologist (RST), 203–204
relationships, 59
relaxation techniques, 59, 79, 168
relaxation training, 150
REM (rapid eye movement)
  brain activity during, 289
  cardiovascular effects, 92–93
  discovery of, 37–38
  dreams during, 27, 87, 109
  identifying, 29–30
  introduction to, 8
  neurotransmitters and, 80–82
  NREM sleep compared to, 86–90
  parasomnias, 89–90, 185
  thermoregulation during, 96
REM density, 110
REM sleep behavior disorder (RBD), 90, 113, 125, 187–189
REM sleep latency, 233

REM sleep rebound, 115
REM-related parasomnias, 185
reproductive problems, 21, 64
respiratory disturbance index (RDI), 234
respiratory system, 21, 63, 91
Respiratory Therapist (RT), 203
rest-and-digest, 94
restless legs syndrome (RLS)
  definition of, 22, 54, 263
  exercise and, 137
  in pregnancy, 124
  symptoms, 179
  in women, 125
restless sleep, 272–273
restoration, 42
retainers, 175
reticular formation (RF), 281
rings, 236
RLS (restless legs syndrome)
  definition of, 22, 54, 263
  exercise and, 137
  in pregnancy, 124
  symptoms, 179
  in women, 125
RN (raphe nuclei), 81, 86, 281
ropinirole, 181
Rosbash, Michael (doctor), 39
rostral fluid shift, 178
routine, 89, 137
RPSGT (Registered Polysomnographic Technologists), 203
RRT (Registered Respiratory Therapist), 203–204
RST (Registered Sleep Technologist), 203–204
RT (Respiratory Therapist), 203

S

SAD (seasonal affective disorder), 53
safety workers, 17
Saper, Clifford (professor), 86–87
saturated fats, 130
schools, 249

SCN (suprachiasmatic nucleus), 82, 97–100, 161
scoring technologist, 204
screen time, 13, 89, 139, 245, 268
seasonal affective disorder (SAD), 53
second-generation medications, 83
sedative, 133
selective attention, 57
selective serotonin reuptake inhibitors (SSRI), 115
sensitivity, 235
sensory experiences, 106–108
serotonin, 81, 283
sex difference, 10
sexsomnia, 185
sexual behaviors, 185
sexuality, 104–105
shift work sleep disorder, 54, 160–161, 163–165
shift workers, 132
short sleep, 128
short-acting hypnotics, 83
shortness of breath, 63
short-term countermeasures, 70–71
SIDS (sudden infant death syndrome), 137, 265
Siegel, Jerome (doctor), 36
single-use device, 226
sixty cycle interference, 221
skin conditions, 263
Sleep and Wakefulness (Kleitman), 36
sleep architecture, 56, 122
sleep attacks, 85, 153
sleep centers, 26, 197–207
sleep cycle, 50, 88–89, 97–100, 233
sleep debt, 20, 46–47
sleep deprivation
  avoiding, 70–73
  economic impact of, 69–70
  impact of, 21, 56–60
  mitigating effects of, 59–60
  modern practices and, 16
  sleep loss compared to, 45
  symptoms, 20
  types of and warning signs, 20–21, 47–52, 129–130

About the Author

Clete A. Kushida, M.D., Ph.D. is a neurologist, division chief and medical director of Stanford Sleep Medicine, associate chair and professor of Psychiatry and Behavioral Sciences at the Stanford University Medical Center, and director of the Stanford Human Sleep Research Laboratory. Dr. Kushida received a B.A.S. degree in the biological sciences and psychology at Stanford University, a M.S. degree in biological sciences at Stanford University, and M.D. and Ph.D. degrees at the University of Chicago. He completed an internal medicine internship at the University of Hawaii, a neurology residency at the University of California, San Diego, and a sleep medicine fellowship at Stanford University.

Dr. Kushida was the inaugural president of the World Sleep Society, past president of the World Sleep Federation, past president of the American Academy of Sleep Medicine, past president of the Associated Professional Sleep Societies board of directors, and founding president of the California Sleep Society. Dr. Kushida has conducted basic and clinical sleep research since 1977, and he served as principal investigator for numerous large federally and industry sponsored studies. He served as chair of the Standards of Practice Committee of the American Academy of Sleep Medicine, and founding chair of both the International Sleep Medicine Practice Recommendations Committee and the International Sleep Research Training Program of the World Sleep Society.

Dr. Kushida has authored or edited over 350 publications and ten books, including serving as editor-in-chief of the largest publication on the field of sleep to date, the *Encyclopedia of Sleep and Circadian Rhythms* (2nd edition, 6 volumes, 454 chapters, 827 authors). He also serves as editor-in-chief of the journal *Sleep Science and Practice*. Dr. Kushida is a past recipient of the highest professional awards in the field of sleep medicine: the American Academy of Sleep Medicine's Nathaniel Kleitman Distinguished Service Award and (twice) the World Sleep Society's Distinguished Service Award.

Dedication

To my wife Shirley, and my sons Caelus and Aetius, who inspire me to be a better person.

Author's Acknowledgments

I am grateful for the assistance of Sarah Sypniewski, Leah Michael, Elizabeth Stilwell, and Amy Handy with the construction of this book. I am deeply indebted to the pioneers of the field of sleep, William C. Dement, Christian Guilleminault, Sonia Ancoli-Israel, Chris Gillin, and Allan Rechtschaffen, who served as my mentors through various stages of my career. Lastly, I want to thank Laura Roberts, Indy Singh, Cindy Tse, Ruch Kumbhani, Mirna Godoy, Tai Mau, Oscar Carrillo, and Jerry Aparece whom I can always count on for support at Stanford. I am fortunate to have had and continue to have terrific collaborators, colleagues, faculty members, coworkers, staff, fellows, research sponsors and coordinators, and trainees over the years.

Publisher's Acknowledgments

Associate Editor: Elizabeth Stilwell
Project Manager: Leah Michael
Copy Editor: Amy Handy
Technical Editor: Sharon Keenan

Production Editor: Saikarthick Kumarasamy
Cover Image: © Antonio Guillem/Shutterstock